POCKET GUIDE
Clinical

Sarah DC
coninck .

Commissioning Editor: Laurence Hunter
Project Development Manager: Janice Urquhart
Project Manager: Nancy Arnott
Designer: George Ajayi

POCKET GUIDE TO
Clinical
Examination

THIRD EDITION

Owen Epstein MB BCh FRCP
Consultant Physician and Gastroenterologist,
Royal Free Hospital NHS Trust, London, UK

G. David Perkin BA MB FRCP
Consultant Neurologist, Regional Neurosciences Centre,
Charing Cross Hospital, London, UK

John Cookson MD FRCP
Professor of Medical Education, Hull York Medical School,
University of York, York, UK
University of Hull, Hull, UK

David P. de Bono (deceased)

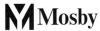

Edinburgh London New York Oxford Philadelphia St Louis Sydney Toronto 2004

MOSBY
An imprint of Elsevier Limited

© 2004, Elsevier Limited. All rights reserved.

The right of Owen Epstein, G. David Perkin and John Cookson to be identified as authors of this work has been asserted by them in accordance with the Copyright, Designs and Patents Act 1988

Second edition 1997
Third edition 2004
  Reprinted 2005, 2006

ISBN 0 7234 3230 9

British Library Cataloguing in Publication Data
A catalogue record for this book is available from the British Library

Library of Congress Cataloging in Publication Data
A catalog record for this book is available from the Library of Congress

Notice

ELSEVIER your source for books,
journals and multimedia
in the health sciences
www.elsevierhealth.com

Working together to grow
libraries in developing countries

www.elsevier.com | www.bookaid.org | www.sabre.org

ELSEVIER   BOOK AID International   Sabre Foundation

The Publisher's policy is to use **paper manufactured from sustainable forests**

Printed in Spain

Preface

The third edition of *Pocket Guide to Clinical Examination* builds on its reputation as a handy reference to the parent book in this series, *Clinical Examination*, 3rd edn. The pocket book contains the core information necessary to take a thorough history and conduct a full physical examination. Like the parent textbook, this pocket guide is richly illustrated in full colour and includes numerous icon boxes which both summarise important information and provide a framework for quick revision. The book is designed to be easily portable, and this third edition contains more content and is designed to be more durable than its predecessor.

O. E.   London

Contents

1.
Medical Record, Medical History and Interviewing Technique

Before setting out to learn about clinical examination, it is important to know how to write up a full medical record. The initial record will include a detailed history and examination as well as plans for investigation and treatment.

PROBLEM-ORIENTATED MEDICAL RECORD (POMR)

The POMR provides a framework for standardising the structure of follow-up notes (Fig. 1.1); this stresses changes in the patient's symptoms and signs and the evolution of clinical assessment and management plans. The POMR also provides a flow sheet that records sequential changes in clinical and biochemical measurements.

The history

The history guides the patient through a series of questions designed to build a profile of the individual and his or her problems. By the end of the first interview you should have a good understanding of the

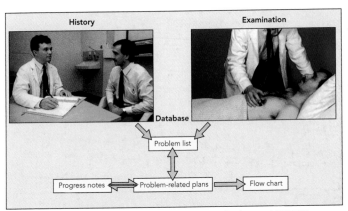

Fig. 1.1 Structure of the problem-orientated medical record (POMR).

patient's personality, social habits and clinical problems. You will have considered a differential diagnosis that may explain the patient's symptoms.

The medical history involves a series of questions ranging from the presenting complaint to the social history, education, employment history, personal habits, travel, home circumstances, family history and review of the major systems.

The examination

The examination may confirm or refute a diagnosis suspected from the history and by adding this information to the database you will be able to construct a more accurate problem list.

Patient's name:		Hospital No:		
No	active problems	date	inactive problems	date
1	jaundice (Jan '02)	9/1/02		
2	anorexia (Dec '02)	9/1/02		
3	weight loss	9/1/02		
4	recurrent rectal bleeding	9/1/02		
5	smoking (since 1980)	9/1/02		
6	unemployed (Nov '01)	9/1/02		
7	stutter	9/1/02		
8			duodenal ulcer (1986)	9/1/02
9				
10				

Fig. 1.2 Problem list entered on 9 January 2002.

Setting up the problem list (Fig. 1.2)

Divide the problems into those that are active (or require active management) and those that are inactive (problems that have resolved or require no action but may be important at some stage in the patient's management).

Your entries into the problem list may include established diagnoses (e.g. ulcerative colitis), symptoms (e.g. dyspnoea), physical signs (e.g. ejection systolic murmur), laboratory tests (e.g. anaemia), psychological and social history (e.g. depression, unemployment, parental or marital problems) or special risk factors (e.g. smoking, alcohol or narcotic abuse). The problem list is designed to accommodate change; consequently, it is not necessary to delete an entry once a higher level of diagnosis (or understanding) is reached. The list should be under constant review to ensure that the entries are accurate and up to date.

Initial problem-related plans

By constructing the problem list so it should be reasonably easy to develop a management plan by considering four headings:

- **Diagnostic tests (Dx)** Write differential next to each problem. Construct a logical flow of investigations by considering bedside tests, side ward tests, plain radiographs, ultrasound, blood tests and specialised imaging examinations.
- **Monitoring tests (Mx)** Consider whether a particular problem can be monitored. Document the appropriate tests and the frequency with which they should be performed.
- **Treatment (Rx)** If drug treatment is indicated, note the drug and dosage.
- **Education (Ed)** Patients are able to cope better with their illness if they understand its nature, its likely course and the effect of treatment.

Progress notes

The POMR provides a disciplined and standardised structure to follow-up notes:

- **Subjective (S)** Record any change in the patient's symptoms.
- **Objective (O)** Record any change in physical signs and investigations that may influence diagnosis, monitoring or treatment.
- **Assessment (A)** Comment on whether the information has confirmed or altered your assessment plans.
- **Plans (P)** Consider whether any modification of the original plan is needed.

Flow charts

A flow sheet is convenient for recording these data in a format that, at a glance, provides a summary of trends and progress (Fig. 1.3). Graphs may be equally revealing (Fig. 1.4).

Date	9.1.02	11.1.02	13.1.02	14.1.02	7.2.02	14.2.02
Tests						
Bilirubin (<17)	233	190	130		28	10
AST (<40)	1140	830	500		52	23
ALT (<45)	1600	650	491		61	31
Albumin (35–45)	41	40	41		42	43
Pro-time (s)	14/12	14/12	13/12	discharged	13/12	12/12
Haemoglobin (11.5–16.2)	12.1	12.3	12.1		12.2	12.6
Blood urea (3.5–6.5)	3.1	4.2	4.8		6.0	6.2
Blood glucose (3.5–6.5)	5.5	6.8	5.0		5.6	6.0
Hepatitis screen			IgM Hep A +ve			
Cholesterol (3.5–6.8)			8.1			8.4

Fig. 1.3 Example of a flow sheet.

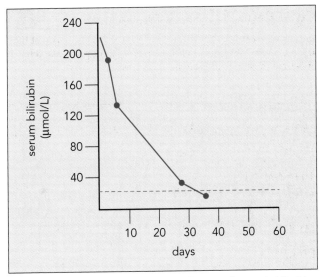

Fig. 1.4 Example of the use of a graph to illustrate changes in bilirubin levels following acute type A hepatitis.

CONFIDENTIALITY

Clinical notes contain confidential information and it is important that you protect this confidentiality. Ensure that there is control over access to the medical record and that only individuals directly involved in the patient's care read or write in the notes.

INTERVIEWING TECHNIQUES AND HISTORY-TAKING

During the interview, you will use a combination of open-ended and closed questions.

Before considering the formal stages of history-taking, you should plan for an optimal setting in which to conduct the interview.

THE INTERVIEW

If possible, you should find a quiet room in which to conduct the interview. Arrange the patient's seat close to yours, rather than confronting him or her across a desk.

Yourself

The white coat and respectful personal presentation are part of our medical culture and are important in establishing the 'role-play' that underlies the medical interview.

Initial approach

Begin by asking the patient to outline the problem by using an open-ended question. Summarise the patient's comments.

The history

HISTORY OF THE PRESENTING COMPLAINT(S)

There is a useful framework for developing a series of questions to follow-up from the initial open-ended question. Symptoms from an organ system have a typical location and character. Establish the location of the symptom, its mode of onset, its progression or regression and aggravating or relieving factors.

For the assessment of pain, use the framework shown in the box.

 Symptoms and signs
Four fundamental questions you are trying to extract for the history

- From which organ(s) do the symptoms arise?
- What is the likely cause?
- Are there any predisposing or risk factors?
- Are there any complications?

SOCIAL HISTORY

Enquire about schooling, employment (past and present), social skills, friends and relationships with partners and families.

EMPLOYMENT HISTORY

Enquire about working conditions as this may be of critical importance if there is suspicion of exposure to an occupational hazard.

DRUG HISTORY

Ask about non-prescription medicines: NSAIDs commonly cause dyspepsia, codeine-containing analgesics cause constipation and antihistamines may cause drowsiness. Ask about and list any drug allergies.

Ask the patient about the use of illicit drugs.

TOBACCO CONSUMPTION

Ask patients what form of tobacco they consume and for how long they have been smoking. If they previously smoked, when did they stop and for how long did they abstain?

ALCOHOL CONSUMPTION

Alcohol history is often inaccurate and the tendency is to underestimate intake. Calculate the amount in units. Certain questions may reveal dependency without asking the patient to specify consumption. Ask about early morning nausea, vomiting and tremulousness, which are typical features of dependency. Does the patient have days without alcohol?

FOREIGN TRAVEL

Ask the patient if he or she has been abroad recently. If so, determine the countries visited and the levels of hygiene maintained.

Symptoms and signs
Units of alcohol equivalents

1 unit is equal to:
- 1/2 a pint of beer
- 1 glass of sherry
- 1 glass of wine
- 1 standard measure of spirits

Risk factors
Travel-related risks

Viral diseases
- hepatitis A, B and E
- yellow fever
- rabies
- polio

Bacterial diseases
- salmonella
- shigella
- enteropathogenic *Escherichia coli*

- cholera
- meningitis
- tetanus
- Lyme disease

Parasite and protozoan diseases
- malaria
- schistosomiasis
- trypanosomiasis
- amoebiasis

HOME CIRCUMSTANCES
- Does the patient live alone? Are there any support systems provided by the community or the family?
- Can the patient attend to personal needs such as bathing, shaving and cooking?
- What effects will the patient's illness have on the financial status of the family?

Family history

Did any family members die at a relatively young age and, if so, from what cause. When there is suspicion of a familial disorder (e.g. Huntington's disease), it is helpful to construct a family tree (Fig. 1.5) If the pattern of inheritance suggests a recessive trait, ask whether the parents were related.

Differential diagnosis
Common disorders expressed in families

- Hyperlipidaemia (ischaemic heart disease)
- Diabetes mellitus
- Hypertension
- Myopia
- Alcoholism
- Depression
- Osteoporosis
- Cancer (bowel, ovarian, breast)

Systems review

Develop a routine that helps to avoid missing out a particular system.

CARDIOVASCULAR SYSTEM
- Chest pain
- Dyspnoea
- Ankle swelling
- Palpitations.

RESPIRATORY SYSTEM
- Cough
- Haemoptysis
- Wheezing
- Pain.

GASTROINTESTINAL SYSTEM
- Change in weight
- Abdominal pain
- Vomiting
- Flatulence and heart burn
- Dysphagia
- Bowel habit.

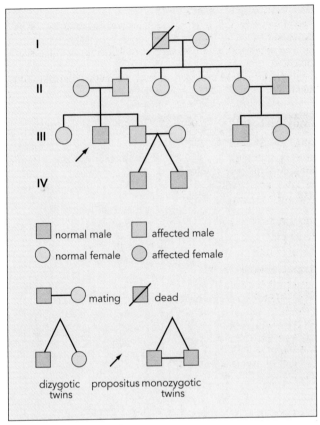

Fig. 1.5 A standard family tree.

GENITOURINARY SYSTEM

- Frequency
  Summarise the findings as a ratio: $\dfrac{\text{Day}}{\text{Night}} = \dfrac{6-8}{0-1}$

- Pain
- Altered bladder control
- Menstruation
- Sexual activity.

NERVOUS SYSTEM

- Headache
- Loss of consciousness
- Dizziness and vertigo
- Speech and related functions
- Memory

CRANIAL NERVE SYMPTOMS
- Vision
- Diplopia
- Facial numbness
- Deafness
- Oropharyngeal dysphagia
- Limb motor or sensory symptoms
- Loss of coordination

ENDOCRINE HISTORY
- Diabetes mellitus (polydipsia, polyuria)
- Thyroid

MUSCULOSKELETAL SYSTEM
- Bone or joint pain?
- Swelling, tenderness redness?
- Single joint or more diffuse?

SKIN
- Rashes?
- Itching?
- Chemicals or cosmetics?

Particular problems

THE PATIENT WITH DEPRESSION OR DEMENTIA
Patients with dementia initially retain some insight and in particular may have reasonable grasp of distant events. Characteristic of Alzheimer's dementia is loss of insight and failure to recognise memory loss. This contrasts with senile dementias in which the patient is often concerned at their memory loss. Involve family, friends and carers in the assessment.

 Examination of elderly people
History-taking

There are special problems when recording a history from elderly patients. Consider the following.

Hearing loss
- Common in the elderly
- May be helped by hearing aid
- Important to speak clearly and slowly
- Face the patient and avoid extraneous sound
- If necessary, write questions in bold letters

Visual handicap
- Cataracts, glaucoma and macular degeneration are common in the elderly

Examination of elderly people
History-taking – *(cont'd)*

- Ensure the room is well lit
- Engage an assistant or carer to help patients move in and out of the consulting room and examination area

Dementia
- Often occurs in patients who appear physically fit
- Forgetfulness, repetition and inappropriate answers characterise responses
- Family members, friends and carers often note the development of dementia

Important aspects of a history from elderly patients include:

- State of the domestic environment and general living conditions
- Provision of community and social services
- Family support structures
- Economic status and pension provision
- Mobility (at home and in the local environment)
- Detailed drug history and compliance
- Provision of laundry services
- Legal will

Review
The history

- Welcome
- Note the patient's body language
- Begin with an open-ended question
- Take a history of the presenting complaint(s); use closed-questions to answer the following:
  - which organ system?
  - likely cause?
  - predisposing factors?
  - complications
- Social history
- Medical history
- Education
- Employment
- Medicines, drugs and tobacco
- Alcohol consumption
- Foreign travel
- Home circumstances
- Family history
- Systems review
  - cardiovascular
  - respiratory
  - gastrointestinal
  - genitourinary
  - nervous
  - endocrine
  - musculoskeletal
  - skin and hair

2.
The General Examination

The examination really begins from the moment you set eyes on the patient. Facial expression, tone of voice and body attitude may signal depression, even if the patient does not complain of feeling depressed.

The formal physical examination follows on from the history and calls on your major senses of sight, touch and hearing. Inspection, palpation, percussion and auscultation form the foundation of the physical examination and this formula is repeated each time you examine an organ system.

The physical examination begins with a general examination and is followed by examination of the skin, head and neck, heart and lungs, abdominal organs, musculoskeletal and neurological systems.

GENERAL EXAMINATION: FIRST IMPRESSIONS

At the first encounter, decide whether the patient looks well or not and whether there is any striking physical abnormality. Observe the posture, gait and character of the stride. You should quickly recognise the slow shuffling gait and 'pill rolling' tremor of Parkinson's disease or the unsteady broad-based gait of the ataxic patient. Patients with proximal muscle weakness may have difficulty rising from the waiting room chair and their gait may have a waddling appearance. Take note if the patient walks with a stick or other physical support.

Short stature may reflect constitutional shortness, a distinct genetic syndrome or the consequence of intrauterine, childhood or adolescent growth retardation.

Symptoms and signs
Observation of general appearance

- Does the patient look comfortable or distressed?
- Is the patient well or ill?
- Is there a recognisable syndrome?
- Is the patient well nourished?
- Is the patient well hydrated?

Posture may provide helpful information. Patients with acute pancreatitis find some relief lying with knees drawn towards the chest. Patients with peritonitis lie motionless, as any abdominal wall movement causes intense pain. In acute pericarditis, the patient finds modest relief by sitting forward; in left ventricular failure, patients breathe more easily when lying propped up on 3 or 4 pillows (orthopnoea).

FORMAL EXAMINATION

The examination requires full exposure.

Begin with a global inspection of overall appearance. When inspecting the face, you might be struck by a single sign such as a red eye or the characteristic facies associated with discrete syndromes.

THE EYE

 Symptoms and signs
Quick testing of visual acuity

- Assess ability of each eye to read newspaper print
- Pinhole test
- Snellen chart

 Differential diagnosis
Main causes of red eye

- Conjunctivitis (infective, allergic, toxic)
- Keratitis (infective, foreign body, sicca syndrome)
- Acute closed angle glaucoma
- Iritis
- Reiter's syndrome

 Symptoms and signs
Penlight inspection of the red eye

- Does the pupil react to light?
- Is the pupil smaller than expected or pinpoint?
- Is there a purulent discharge?
- What is the pattern of the redness?
- Is there a corneal 'white spot'?
- Is there hypopyon or hyphema?

RECOGNISABLE SYNDROMES AND FACIES

Genetic or chromosomal syndromes that may present to clinicians caring for adults include Down's syndrome, Turner's syndrome, Marfan's syndrome, tuberous sclerosis, albinism, the fragile X chromosome Peutz–Jeghers syndrome, Waardenburg's syndrome, familial hypercholesterolaemia and neurofibromatosis.

Symptoms and signs
Down's syndrome (trisomy 21)

- Facies – oblique orbital fissures, epicanthic folds, small ears, flat nasal bridge, protruding tongue, Brushfield's spots on iris
- Short stature
- Hands – single palmar crease, curved little finger, short hands
- Heart disease (endocardial cushion defects)
- Gap between first and second toes
- Learning difficulties

ENDOCRINE SYNDROMES

It is practical to consider the examination of the endocrine glands in the context of the overall general examination.

Distinct clinical syndromes occur in diseases of the thyroid, parathyroid, adrenal and pituitary glands.

Clinical examination of the thyroid gland

Questions to ask
Hyperthyroidism

- Have you lost weight recently?
- Has your appetite changed (e.g. increased)?
- Have you noticed a change in bowel habit (e.g. increased)?
- Have you noticed a recent change in heat tolerance?
- Do you suffer from excessive sweating?
- Does your heart race or palpitate?
- Have you noticed a change in mood?

Symptoms and signs
Hyperthyroidism

- Weight loss, increased appetite
- Recent onset of heat intolerance
- Agitation, nervousness
- Hot, sweaty palms
- Fine peripheral tremor
- Bounding peripheral pulses
- Tachycardia, atrial fibrillation
- Lid retraction and lid lag
- Goitre, with or without overlying bruit
- Brisk tendon reflexes

GRAVES' DISEASE

 Symptoms and signs
Graves' disease (autoimmune hyperthyroidism)

- Diffuse goitre with audible bruit
- Pretibial myxoedema, finger clubbing
- Onycholysis (Plummer's nails)
- Lid retraction, lid lag
- Proptosis, exophthalmos
- Conjunctival oedema (chemosis)

HYPOTHYROIDISM

Hypothyroidism presents insidiously; the diagnosis may be readily apparent on general examination.

 Questions to ask
Hypothyroidism

- Has your weight changed?
- Has your bowel habit changed (e.g. constipation)?
- Is your hair falling out?
- Have you noticed a change in weather preference (e.g. cold intolerance)?
- Has there been a change in your voice (e.g. hoarse)?
- Do you suffer from pain in your hands (e.g. carpal tunnel syndrome)?

Symptoms and signs
Hypothyroidism

- Constipation, weight gain
- Hair loss
- Angina pectoris
- Hoarse, croaky voice
- Dry flaky skin
- Balding and loss of eyebrows (beginning laterally)
- Bradycardia
- Xanthelasmas (hyperlipidaemia)
- Goitre (especially with iodine deficiency)
- Effusions (pericardial or pleural)
- Delayed relaxation phase of tendon reflexes
- Carpal tunnel syndrome

Differential diagnosis
Hypothyroidism

Congenital
- Congenital absence
- Inborn errors of thyroxine metabolism

Acquired
- Iodine deficiency (endemic goitre)
- Autoimmune thyroiditis (Hashimoto's disease)
- Postradiotherapy for hyperthyroidism
- Postsurgical thyroidectomy
- Antithyroid drugs (e.g. carbimazole)
- Pituitary tumours and granulomas

Hyperparathyroidism

Hyperparathyroidism is usually detected by finding an abnormally high serum calcium level on routine blood testing. The clinical syndrome may be difficult to recognise, because the symptoms ('moans') dominate the signs ('stones and bones'). The patient complains of tiredness and lethargy, excessive thirst and symptoms of increased urine output. There may be profound changes in the mental state and, in severe cases, drowsiness and even coma may occur. Renal stones are common and the patient may present with severe acute unilateral abdominal pain radiating towards the groin. There may be proximal muscle weakness (due to a myopathy), a thin opaque ring around the limbus of the cornea, and bone pain or radiological evidence of hyperparathyroidism.

Hypoparathyroidism

Surgical damage or removal of three of four parathyroid glands during neck surgery (usually thyroidectomy) is the most common cause of hypoparathyroidism. The serum calcium level is low (in the presence of a normal serum albumin). The major symptoms of acute hypoparathyroidism are paraesthesiae around the mouth, fingers and toes. Abnormal nerve and muscle irritability can be elicited with Chvostek's (Fig. 2.1) and Trousseau's signs (Fig. 2.2).

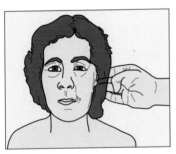

Fig. 2.1 Chvostek's sign. Tap over the facial nerve in front of the ear, this causes a momentary twitch of the corner of the mouth on the same side as the irritable facial muscles contract.

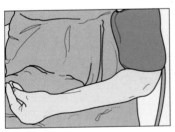

Fig. 2.2 Trousseau's sign. Inflate a sphygmomanometer cuff to above systolic pressure. Within approximately 4 min, there is characteristic 'carpopedal' spasm of the hand. There is opposition of the thumb, extension of the interphalangeal joints and flexion of the metacarpophalangeal joints. This posture reverses spontaneously when the cuff is deflated.

Biochemical assessment of thyroid function

T_4 has a number of important metabolic effects and over- and underactivity results in characteristic clinical syndromes that may readily be recognised. Diagnosis of hyperthyroidism is confirmed by measuring the serum levels of T_4 and T_3, whereas in hypothyroidism the serum TSH level is elevated and T_4 is subnormal.

Hyperadrenalism (Cushing's syndrome)

Excessive glucocorticoids (either endogenous or exogenous) cause a significant change in body appearance which can be readily recognised as Cushing's syndrome.

Differential diagnosis
Hyperadrenalism

- Iatrogenic, exogenous steroids
- Bilateral adrenal hyperplasia
- Benign autonomous adrenal adenoma
- Malignant adrenal adenocarcinoma
- Nonmetastatic tumour effect (e.g. lung cancer producing ACTH-like peptide)
- Alcoholism causing pseudo-Cushing's syndrome

Symptoms and signs
Cushing's syndrome

- Round, moon-shaped, plethoric facies
- Hirsutes
- Acne
- Hypertension
- Buffalo hump on neck (fatty deposit)
- Central distribution of fat
- Proximal muscle weakness and wasting
- Purple skin striae

Hypoadrenalism and Addison's disease

In acute adrenal failure, the clinical features may be nonspecified and puzzling. The most helpful physical sign is the profound drop in blood pressure when the patient changes position from lying to standing (postural hypotension).

Symptoms and signs
Presenting features of acute adrenal (Addisonian) crisis

- Profound dehydration, postural hypotension, shock
- Severe nausea and vomiting associated with unexplained weight loss
- Acute abdominal pain
- Unexplained hypoglycaemia
- Unexplained fever
- Hyponatraemia, hyperkalaemia, uraemia hypercalcaemia, eosinophilia
- Hyperpigmentation or vitiligo

Syndromes associated with overproduction of pituitary hormones

ACROMEGALY

Acidophil (or more rarely chromophobe) tumours of the anterior pituitary may cause inappropriate release of growth hormone.

Symptoms and signs
Acromegaly

- Coarse, prominent facial features
- Prognathid jaw
- Prominent nose and forehead
- Thickened lips and large tongue
- 'Spade-shaped' hands
- Excessive sweating and greasy skin
- Kyphosis
- Hypertension
- Bitemporal hemianopia develops
- Carpal tunnel syndrome
- Impaired glucose tolerance

HYPERPROLACTINAEMIA

The syndromes associated with the overproduction of prolactin may be dominated by either the effect of the prolactin or the destructive effect of the pituitary tumour.

Syndromes associated with pituitary hypofunction

HYPOPITUITARISM

The clinical features progress in a characteristic sequence. Growth and luteinising hormone failure occurs first, followed by FSH and TSH and finally ACTH.

Impaired ADH secretion causes a typical syndrome known as cranial diabetes insipidus. Patients have inappropriate polyuria and produce a dilute urine, even when deprived of water for prolonged periods.

Symptoms and signs
Hypopituitarism

Women
- amenorrhoea, infertility
- vaginal atrophy, dyspareunia
- atrophic breasts
- loss of axillary and pubic hair

Men
- loss of libido or impotence, infertility
- soft atrophic testes and loss of secondary sexual characteristics

- TSH deficiency, mild to moderate hypothyroidism
- ACTH deficiency – weakness
  – postural hypotension
  – pallor
  – hypoglycaemia

NUTRITION

Assessment of nutrition

Weigh the patient and measure the height. This provides useful baseline information, as standard growth charts are available to help you judge whether the patient falls within the normal range of weight for height (Fig. 2.3). Body mass index (BMI) is the preferred method for assessing weight, as it considers both weight and height. This is calculated from the formula:

$$\frac{\text{height (m)}}{\text{weight (kg)}^2}$$

The normal BMI range is 20–25.

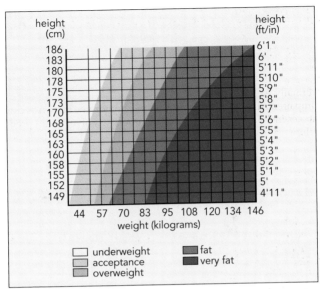

Fig. 2.3 Chart indicating height and weight norms in adults.

When the patient is exposed during the course of the physical examination, evaluate whether the patient is, unusually thin or overweight. Weight loss and 'wasting' are suggested by indrawing of the cheeks and unusual prominence of the cheek-bones, head of humerus and major joints, the rib cage and bony landmarks of the pelvis. Hypoalbuminaemia may cause white nails (leukonychia), and loss of capillary osmotic pressure results in pedal oedema. Iron deficiency may cause spooning of the nails (koilonychia). Other features of nutritional deficiency include inflammation and cracks at the angle of the mouth (angular stomatitis), a smooth tongue lacking in papillae (atrophic glossitis) and skin rashes (e.g. pellagra).

MIDARM MUSCLE CIRCUMFERENCE
This measurement provides estimate of muscle and fat status (Fig. 2.4).

TRICEPS SKINFOLD THICKNESS
In adults, the skin overlying the triceps muscle can be lifted and subcutaneous tissue can be distinguished from the underlying muscle bulk. This fold of skin and subcutaneous tissue (the fatfold) provides an indirect assessment of fat stores (Fig. 2.5)

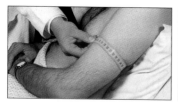

Fig. 2.4 Measurement of the midarm muscle circumference.

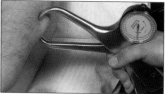

Fig. 2.5 Measurement of the triceps skinfold thickness.

CLINICAL ASSESSMENT OF VITAMIN STATUS

 Symptoms and signs
Vitamin deficiency syndromes

Fat-soluble vitamin	Clinical features of deficiency
A	Dry eyes and skin, night blindness, corneal thinning (keratomalacia)
D	Proximal muscle weakness, bone pain, osteomalacia
K	Easy bleeding, bruising

 Symptoms and signs
Water-soluble vitamin deficiency

B1 (thiamine)
- Wet beriberi
  - peripheral vasodilation
  - high output cardiac failure
  - oedema
- Dry beriberi
  - sensory and motor peripheral neuropathy
- Wernicke's encephalopathy
  - ataxia, nystagmus, lateral rectus palsy
  - altered mental state
- Korsakoff's psychosis
  - retrograde amnesia, impaired learning
  - confabulation

B2 (riboflavin)
- Inflamed oral mucous membranes
- Angular stomatitis
- Glossitis, normocytic anaemia

Symptoms and signs
Water-soluble vitamin deficiency – *(cont'd)*

B3 (niacin)
- Pellagra
- Dermatitis (photosensitive)
- Diarrhoea
- Dementia

B6 (pyridoxine)
- Peripheral neuropathy
- Sideroblastic anaemia

B12
- Megaloblastic, macrocytic anaemia
- Glossitis
- Subacute combined degeneration of the cord

Folic acid
- Megaloblastic, macrocytic anaemia
- Glossitis

C
- Scurvy
  - perifollicular haemorrhage
  - bleeding gums, skin purpura
  - bleeding into muscles and joints
- Anaemia
- Osteoporosis

CLINICAL ASSESSMENT OF HYDRATION

Dehydration rapidly provokes thirst, the first clinical symptom of dehydration. Physical signs of dehydration are usually only apparent with moderate to severe dehydration. Inspect the tongue and note whether the mucosa is wet and glistening.

With moderate dehydration, the eyes may appear sunken into the orbits; the pulse rate may increase to compensate for intravascular volume loss. Blood pressure falls in hypovolaemic patients and the demonstration of postural hypotension is a cardinal sign of significant intravascular fluid loss. In addition, the capillary refill time can be used to assess the circulation effects of volume depletion.

With marked dehydration skin turgor is lost. This can be demonstrated by gently pinching a fold of skin, holding the fold for a few moments and letting it go. In dehydration the skinfold only slowly returns back to normal.

Symptoms and signs
Measurement of postural change in blood pressure

- Lie the patient supine for 2 min
- Record pulse rate and blood pressure in supine position
- Ask the patient to stand upright
- Wait 1 min
- Measure standing heart rate and blood pressure at 1 and 3 min
- Heart rate normally increase by 8–12 beats/min
- Systolic blood pressure drops by 3–4 mmHg
- Diastolic blood pressure increases by 3–7 mmHg
- Postural hypotension when systolic drops by 20 mmHg and/or diastolic by 10 mmHg

Symptoms and signs
Measuring the capillary refill time

- Patient's hand placed level with the heart
- Distal phalanx of the middle finger compressed for 5 s
- Release pressure
- Measure time to regain normal colour (refill time)
- Normal filling time is 2–3 s (2–4 s in the elderly)

CLINICAL ASSESSMENT OF SHOCK

Differential diagnosis
Shock

- Hypovolaemic shock
  - GI bleeding
  - trauma
  - ruptured aneurysm
  - burns
  - haemorrhagic pancreatitis
  - fractures (e.g. neck of femur)
  - diarrhoea and vomiting
- Cardiogenic shock
  - acute myocardial infarction
  - acute arrhythmias
  - acute rupture of a valve cusp
  - pericardial tamponade
- Distributive shock
  - gram-negative sepsis
  - toxic shock syndrome
  - anaphylaxis
  - Addisonian crisis
  - spinal cord/major brain injury

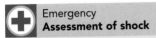

**Emergency
Assessment of shock**

- Early rise in pulse rate
- Reduced pulse volume/pulse pressure
- Orthostatic hypotension
- Recumbent hypotension
- Cool pale peripheries
- Delayed capillary filling time
- Dry mucous membranes
- Oliguria
- Altered mental state
- Signs of metabolic acidosis

COLOUR

Pallor

The palpebral conjunctiva is normally a healthy red colour but, in anaemia, it appears a pale pink.

Pallor is an unreliable sign in cold or shocked patients because peripheral vasoconstriction causes skin and conjunctival pallor even when not associated with blood loss.

Plethora

This refers to a ruddy 'weather beaten' facial appearance where the skin has an unusually red or bluish (cyanosed) appearance. Facial plethora is usually caused by an abnormally high haemoglobin concentration (polycythaemia). This is usually caused by chronic cyanotic lung disease in which hypoxia stimulates erythropoietin.

Polycythaemia rubra vera is a myeloproliferative disorder that causes very high haemoglobin levels. Plethora occurs in the absence of hypoxic cyanosis. The conjunctiva has a characteristic 'plum' colour and on fundoscopy the increased blood viscosity causes the venules to assume a thickened 'sausage-shaped' appearance.

Cyanosis

Cyanosis refers to a bluish or purplish discoloration of the skin or mucous membranes caused by excessive amounts of reduced haemoglobin in blood. In peripheral cyanosis, the extremities are cyanosed but the tongue retains a healthy pink colour. This is caused by any condition resulting in slowing of the peripheral circulation, allowing more time for the extraction of oxygen from haemoglobin. A reduction in arterial oxygen saturation results in central cyanosis. The extremities are cyanosed and the tongue and mucous membranes also have a bluish or purple discoloration. Central cyanosis may develop in any lung disease in which there is a mismatch between ventilation and perfusion.

Jaundice

The sclera is the most sensitive area for looking for the yellow discoloration of jaundice.

Eating large amounts of carrots or other carotene-containing vegetables or substances causes carotenaemia, which can be confused with jaundice. The yellow discoloration is prominent in the face, palms and soles but, in contrast to jaundice, the sclera remains white.

Pigmentation

In iron overload (haemochromatosis), the skin colour may appear slate grey. In chronic cholestasis (e.g. primary biliary cirrhosis), skin hyperpigmentation may develop, especially over pressure points. A marked increase in pigmentation occurs after bilateral adrenalectomy for adrenal hyperplasia.

OEDEMA

The distribution of excess fluid depends on its underlying cause, the shifting effect of gravity and the capacity of the tissue in which it accumulates. In congestive heart failure, patients often notice marked ankle swelling (dependent oedema), which becomes more noticeable as the day wears on and appears to resolve through the night. At night, the recumbent position causes redistribution of the transcapillary and gravitational forces so that by early morning the oedema is most prominent in the sacral region and appears to have resolved from around the ankles.

Symptoms of oedema

If the oedema is generalised, patients may notice tight-fitting shoes, frank swelling of the legs or an unexplained increase in weight. Symptoms are linked to underlying diseases such as heart failure and liver, kidney, bowel or nutritional disease. Localised oedema may be obvious if there is venous thrombosis, regional lymphatic obstruction or a painful, inflamed area of swelling. Fluid accumulation in the pleural space (hydrothorax or pleural effusion) may cause breathlessness. Ascites may be noticed as an increase in girth, weight gain or the eversion of the umbilicus.

Signs of oedema

Press the ball of your thumb or the tips of your index and middle fingers into the posterior malleolar space and maintain moderate pressure for a few seconds. On removing your thumb or fingers, the finger impression remains imprinted in the skin for a short while before fading as the oedema redistributes.

In the recumbent posture, oedema is less obvious around the ankles and most prominent over the sacrum and lower back. In anasarca, oedema extends to the thighs, scrotum and anterior abdominal wall. Anasarca occurs in hypoproteinaemic states (especially nephrotic syndrome, malnutrition and malabsorption), severe cardia or renal failure and when there is a generalised increase in capillary permeability (e.g. severe allergic reactions).

Localised oedema may occur in deep venous thrombosis of the leg veins. The affected limb becomes swollen and if there is thrombophlebitis and rapid muscle swelling, the calf muscle may be tender to palpation (Homan's sign).

Lymphatic oedema has a high protein content. The swelling is pronounced and on palpation the skin has an indurated, thickened feel. This 'brawny' oedema is the clinical hallmark of lymphoedema.

Ascites is characterised by abdominal distention (especially in the flanks) and, on examination, there is shifting dullness.

MEASURING TEMPERATURE

Temperature may be measured by placing a thermometer under the tongue, in the rectum or under the axilla.

Normal temperature

'Normal' oral temperature is usually considered to be 37°C. Rectal temperature is 0.5°C higher than the mouth; the axilla 0.5°C lower. Remember there are small variations between individuals (which may range from 35.8 to 37.1°C). There is also a distinct diurnal variation: oral temperature is usually about 37°C on waking in the morning, rising to a daytime peak between 6.00 and 10.00 p.m. and falling to a low point between 2.00 and 4.00 a.m. In menstruating women, ovulation is accompanied by a 0.5°C increase in body temperature.

Fig. 2.6 Temperature may be described as intermittent, remittent, persistent or spiking.

Fever

Sequential recording of temperature may show a variety of patterns (Fig. 2.6).

Chills and rigors

High fever may be accompanied by a subjective sensation of chill, which may be accompanied by goose pimples, shivering and chattering of the teeth. As the fever subsides, the defervescence is accompanied by hot sensations and intense sweating.

Dx Differential diagnosis
Rigors

- Biliary sepsis (Charcot's triad)
  - jaundice
  - right hypochondrial pain and tenderness
  - fever and rigors
- Pyelonephritis
- Visceral abscesses (liver, lung, paracolic)
- Malaria

Hypothermia

Patients are pale, the skin feels cold and waxy and the muscles are stiff. Consciousness is depressed, and when the temperature drops to below 27°C, consciousness is lost. A low-reading thermometer is required to establish the baseline temperature.

 Differential diagnosis
Hypothermia

- Environmental exposure
- Hypothyroidism
- Increased cutaneous heat loss – burns, toxic epidermal necrolysis
- Drugs (alcohol, opiates, barbiturates, phenothiazines, lithium)
- Altered thermoregulation (sepsis, hypothalamic disease, spinal cord injury)

EXAMINATION OF THE LYMPHATIC SYSTEM

The lymph nodes

Infected nodes are enlarged and tender (lymphadenitis) and the overlying skin may be red and inflamed. When superficial lymphatic vessels leading to a group of nodes are inflamed (lymphangitis), the channels can be seen as thin red streaks leading from a more distal site of inflammation.

Normal nodes are not palpable. If you feel nodes, assess their size (length and width), consistency (soft, firm, rubbery, hard or craggy), tenderness and mobility to surronding nodes and tissues. Inspect the draining area in an attempt to find a source. Painful, tender nodes usually indicate an infected source that may be hidden from obvious view (e.g. infected cracks between toes). Malignant lymph nodes (either primary or secondary) are not usually tender. Malignant lymph nodes may feel unsually firm or hard and irregular. Fixation to surrounding tissue is highly suspicious of malignancy. Matted glands may occur in tuberculous lymphadenitis.

Often, in the course of routine examination, you will discover one or more small, mobile, nontender 'peasized' lymph nodes. Before embarking on a major exercise to diagnose the cause of the lymphadenopathy, re-examine the node a few weeks later. If there is no change in symptoms and signs or gland size consider the node a relic of a previous illness.

HEAD AND NECK NODES

Examine the nodes encircling the lower face and neck. Palpate the nodes in sequence, starting with the submental group in the midline behind the tip of the mandible. Next, feel for the submandibular nodes midway and along the inner surface of the inferior margin of the mandible. Feel for the tonsillar node at the angle of the jaw, the preauricular nodes immediately in front of the ear, the postauricular nodes over the mastoid process and, finally, the occipital nodes at the base of the skull posteriorly. Follow this examination with palpation of the vertical groups of neck nodes. Feel for the superficial cervical nodes along the body of sternocleidomastoid (Fig. 2.19). The posterior cervical nodes run along the anterior border of trapezius. The deep cervical chain is deep to the long axis of sternocleidomastoid. Conclude the examination by probing the supraclavicular nodes which lie in the area bound by the clavicle inferiorly and the lateral border of sternocleidomastoid medially. A palpable left supraclavicular node (Virchow's node) should always alert you to the possibility of stomach cancer.

EPITROCHLEAR AND AXILLARY NODES

To palpate the epitrochlear node, passively flex the patient's relaxed elbow to a right angle. Feel with your fingers for the epitrochlear nodes which lie in a groove above and posterior to the medial condyle of the humerus. The axillary group includes anterior, posterior, central, lateral and brachial nodes. The technique for examining this region is described in Chapter 8.

INGUINAL AND LEG NODES

The superficial inguinal nodes run in two chains. Palpate the horizontal chain which runs just below the line of the inguinal ligament and the vertical chain which runs along the saphenous vein. Relax the posterior popliteal fossa by passively flexing the knee. Explore the fossa by wrapping the hands around either side of the knee and exploring the fossa with the fingers of both hands.

 Examination of elderly people
Nutrition in the elderly

- Elderly at special risk of nutritional compromise
- Contributory factors
  - socioeconomic
  - inability to shop
  - loneliness
  - loss of smell, taste and teeth

Examination of elderly people
Nutrition in the elderly – *(cont'd)*

- Age-related norms for height, weight, midarm muscle circumference and triceps skinfold thickness unavailable for elderly people
- Nutrition best assessed by careful dietary assessment (using 3rd party to validate information), and the use of haematological and biochemical markers
- Assessment of hydration affected by loss of elastic tissue in skin

Review
Framework for choreographing the physical examination

General examination
- First impression
- Clinical syndromes (including endocrinopathies)
- Nutritional status
- Hydration
- 'Colour'
- Oedema
- Temperature
- Lymphoreticular examination

Skin examination
- Skin inspection
- Palpation
- Description of lesions
- Hair
- Nails

Ears, nose and throat examination
- Inspection of outer ear, drum; test hearing and balance
- Inspection of nose and palpation/percussion of sinuses
- Inspection of lips, teeth, tongue, oral cavity and pharynx, inspection and palpation of salivary glands
- Palpation of regional lymph nodes

Cardiovascular examination
- Hands (splinters, clubbing)
- Pulses
- Blood pressure
- Jugular venous, pressure
- Heart (inspect, palpate, auscultate)
- Lungs (basal crackles, effusions)

Review
Framework for choreographing the physical examination – *(cont'd)*

- Abdomen (liver pulsation)
- Extremities (peripheral circulation, oedema)

Respiratory examination
- Hands (clubbing, cyanosis, CO_2, retention)
- Blood pressure (pulsus paradoxus)
- Neck (JVP, trachea)
- Lungs (inspect, palpate, percuss, auscultate)
- Heart (evidence of cor pulmonale)

Abdominal examination
- Hands (flapping tremor, nails, palms)
- Jaundice and signs of liver failure
- Parotids
- Mouth and tongue
- Chest (gynaecomastia, spiders, upper border of liver)
- Abdomen (inspect, palpate, percuss, auscultate)
- Groins
- Rectal examination

Male genitalia
- Sexual development
- Penis
- Scrotum
- Testes and spermatic cord
- Inguinal region

Female breasts and genitalia
- Sexual development
- Breast (inspection, palpation)
- Vulva (inspection, palpation)
- Vagina (inspection, palpation)
- Uterus and adnexae (palpation)

Musculoskeletal examination
- Proximal and distal muscles (inspection, palpation)
- Large joints
- Small joints
- Spine
- Psychological profile
- Mental status
- Cranial nerves
- Motor and sensory examination (central and peripheral), cerebellar examination
- Autonomic nervous system

3.
Skin, Nails and Hair

SYMPTOMS OF SKIN DISEASE

The history should evaluate possible precipitating factors and determine whether the skin problem is localised or a manifestation of systemic illness.

Questions to ask
Skin history

- Has there been a change in your mood?
- Has your memory deteriorated?
- Do you have difficulty finding the right word in conversation?
- Have you ever become lost while travelling a familiar route?
- Do you have difficulty dressing?
- Was the onset sudden or gradual?
- Is the skin itchy or painful?
- Is there any associated discharge (blood or pus)?
- Where is the problem located?
- Have you recently taken any antibiotics or other drugs?
- Have you used any topical medications?
- Were there any preceding systemic symptoms (fever, sore throat, anorexia, vaginal discharge)?
- Have you travelled abroad recently?
- Were you bitten by insects?
- Any possible exposure to industrial or domestic toxins?
- Any possible contact with sexually transmitted disease or HIV?
- Was there close physical contact with others with skin disorders?

Differential diagnosis
Systemic diseases causing pruritus

- Intrahepatic and extrahepatic biliary obstruction (cholestasis)
- Diabetes mellitus
- Polycythaemia rubra vera
- Chronic renal failure
- Lymphoma (especially Hodgkin's disease)

Hair thinning

Male pattern baldness is common; the patient will note the slow onset of hair loss with the hairline receding from the frontal and temporal scalp and crown.

Questions to ask
Hair history

- Was the hair loss sudden or gradual?
- Does the loss occur only on the scalp or is the body hair involved as well?
- Is the baldness localised or general, symmetrical or asymmetrical?
- Is there a family history of baldness (especially in men)?
- What drugs have you taken recently?
- Any recent illnesses, stress or trauma?
- Are there other systemic symptoms (e.g. symptoms of hypothyroidism)?

Patients complaining of localised alopecia (alopecia areata) may have an autoimmune disease. Severe illness and malnutrition, as well as sudden psychological shock, may be associated with hair loss, which usually recovers once the stress has been resolved.

Abnormal hair growth

Failure to develop axillary and pubic hair at the expected time of puberty should alert you to the possibility of pituitary or gonadal dysfunction.

Abnormal facial hair growth (hirsutism) is distressing in women. There are racial differences: physiological hirsutism is least apparent in Japanese and Chinese women and most apparent in women of Mediterranean, Middle Eastern, Indian and Negroid extraction.

Differential diagnosis
Hirsutism

- Racial variation in hair distribution
- Hormonal imbalance
  - polycystic ovaries
  - ovarian failure or menopause
  - virilising adrenal tumours
- Drugs
  - phenytoin
  - progestogens
  - anabolic steroids
  - ciclosporin

Questions to ask
Hirsutism

- Is there a family history of hirsutism?
- Are your menstrual periods normal or absent (or scanty)?
- Is there a history of primary or secondary infertility?
- Do you experience visual disturbances or headaches (pituitary disease)?
- What medications do you take (e.g. phenytoin, anabolic steroids, progestogens)?

EXAMINATION OF THE SKIN, NAILS AND HAIR

Examining the skin

Examination relies almost entirely on careful inspection.

ABNORMAL SKIN COLOUR

Changes in skin colour occur in jaundice, iron overload, endocrine disorders and albinism. The yellow tinge of jaundice is best observed in good day-light, appearing as yellowing of the sclerae and then as a yellow discoloration on the trunk, arms and legs.

Iron overload (haemosiderosis and haemochromatosis) causes the skin to turn a slate-grey colour. Addison's disease is characterised by darkening of the skin, occurring first in the skin creases of the palms and soles, scars and other skin creases. The mucosa of the mouth and gums also becomes pigmented. Striking pigmentation arises after bilateral adrenalectomy for adrenal hyperplasia (Nelson's syndrome).

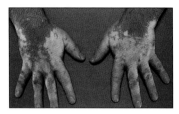

Fig. 3.1 Depigmented skin (vitiligo): white discoloration of brown hand.

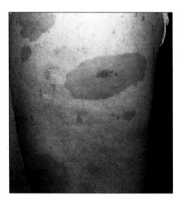

Fig. 3.2 Café au lait patches in neurofibromatosis.

Albinism is an autosomal recessive disorder. The skin and hair are white and the eyes are pink because of a lack of pigmentation of the iris (there may also be nystagmus).

Common localised abnormalities of skin pigmentation include vitiligo (Fig. 3.1) and café au lait spots (Fig. 3.2). When examining a patient, you may notice an erythematous flush in the necklace area which is caused by anxiety. Purpura is the term used for red-purplish lesions of the skin caused by seepage of blood from skin blood vessels. These lesions do not blanch with pressure. If the lesions are small (<5 mm) they are called petechiae, whereas larger lesions are purpura.

LOCALISED SKIN LESIONS

Decide whether the lesion is flat, nodular or fluid-filled. Flat circumscribed changes in colour are termed macules if less than 1 cm, or patches if more than 1 cm. If the lesion is raised and can be palpated, assess whether the mass is a papule, plaque, nodule, tumour or wheal. If a circumscribed elevated lesion is fluctuant and fluid-filled, describe whether it is a vesicle, bulla or pustule (Fig. 3.3).

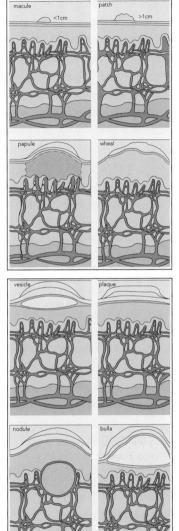

Fig. 3.3 Primary localised skin lesions.

Add to the primary description any secondary characteristics such as superficial erosions, ulceration, crusting, scaling, fissuring, lichenification, atrophy, excoriation, scarring, necrosis or keloid formation.

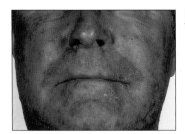

Fig. 3.4 Rosacea: lesions occur on the nose, cheeks and chin.

Compression may be helpful (e.g. demonstration of the characteristic arteriolar dilatation of spider naevi occurring in decompensated liver disease). Inflamed lesions (e.g. cellulitis) are hotter than surrounding tissue, whereas skin overlying a lipoma (subcutaneous fat tumours) is cooler than adjacent tissue.

COMMON SKIN LESIONS
Acne vulgaris
Acne presents with greasy skin, blackheads (comedones), papules, pustules and scars. The disorder affects the face, chest and back. Acne usually subsides in the third decade.

Rosacea
This facial rash usually presents in the fourth decade. Papules and pustules erupt on the forehead, cheeks, bridge of the nose and the chin. The erythematous background highlights the rash (Fig. 3.4). Eye involvement is characterised by grittiness, conjunctivitis and even corneal ulceration.

Drug reactions
Drug reactions may occur within minutes or hours of taking the medication but there may also be delays of up to 2 weeks for the reaction to manifest. It is important to recognise different expressions of drug sensitivity.

 Differential diagnosis
Skin lesions associated with drug sensitivity

- Toxic erythema
- Exfoliative dermatitis
- Urticaria
- Angioneurotic oedema
- Erythema nodosum
- Erythema multiforme
- Fixed drug reaction
- Photosensitive drug reactions
- Pemphigus

Toxic erythema
Profuse eruptions affect most of the body. Red macules appear and overlap and coalesce to give the appearance of diffuse erythema. This condition is most often caused by ampicillin but also by sulphonamides (including co-trimoxazole), phenobarbital and infections.

Exfoliative dermatitis
Also known as erythroderma, this dermatitis is characterised by diffuse erythema and desquamation of the epithelium. Barbiturates, sulphonamides, streptomycin and gold are especially implicated.

Urticaria
Presents with intense itching and localised swellings of the skin that may occur anywhere on the body. Typically, wheals occur that are red at the margins with paler centres.

Erythema nodosum
Symmetrical in distribution, the acute crops of painful, tender, raised red nodules usually affect the extensor surfaces, especially the shins but also the thighs and upper arms (Fig. 3.5). Over 7–10 days, lesions change colour from bright red through shades of purple to a yellowish area of discoloration. Erythema nodosum is caused by vasculitis, and most commonly associated with sulphonamides, oral contraceptives and barbiturates.

 Differential diagnosis
Erythema nodosum

Infections
- Streptococcal infections
- Tuberculosis
- Leprosy
- Syphilis
- Deep fungal diseases

Drugs
- Sulphonamides
- Barbiturates
- Oral contraceptives

Systemic diseases
- Sarcoidosis
- Inflammatory bowel disease

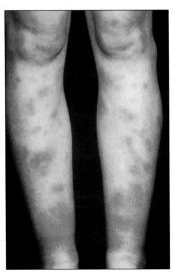

Fig. 3.5 Erythema nodosum: the nodules are raised and tender.

Erythema multiforme
Symmetrical, round (annular) lesions occurring especially on the hands and feet but which may extend more proximally. Central blistering may occur, giving the appearance of 'target' lesions. In severe forms, bullae may appear.

Stevens–Johnson syndrome
This is a severe blistering form of erythema multiforme with blistering and ulceration affecting the mucous membranes of the mouth and often affecting the eyes and nasal and genital mucosa.

Fixed drug eruption
One or more red blotches that may become swollen and even bullous. The rash always recurs in the same anatomical site: usually the mouth, a limb or genital area. Associated especially with phenolphthalein (common in laxatives), sulphonamides, tetracycline and barbiturates.

Photosensitive drug rashes
Occur in sun-exposed areas (face, necklace region and extensor surfaces of limbs). It may appear as erythema, oedema, blistering or an eczematous rash.

Eczema
Acute eczema is characterised by oedema, vesicle formation, exudation (weeping) and crusting. In chronic eczema there are dry,

scaly, hyperkeratotic patches and thickening and fissuring of the skin. The appearance of eczema is often modified because the patient scratches, causing secondary changes such as excoriation and secondary infection.

Discoid (nummular) eczema   This subtype has a well-defined, coin-shaped outline and may be confused with psoriasis. However, nummular eczema tends to occur on the back of the fingers and hands. It also weeps and does not have the characteristic scales typical of psoriasis.

Atopic eczema   Usually presents in infancy, although occasionally presents for the first time in adulthood. The rash is symmetrical, usually starting on the face and migrating to the trunk and limbs.

Contact dermatitis   This is caused by an exogenous irritant. The distribution of the eczema may provide an important clue to the nature of the topical irritant. Jewellery may cause an allergic contact dermatitis; nickel is an important sensitising agent.

Seborrhoeic dermatitis   An eczematous condition occurring in adolescents and young adults. There is erythema and scaling with a symmetrical rash. The scalp is most commonly involved and the condition is distinguished from dandruff by the associated erythema of the skin due to inflammation. Other regions involved include the central areas of the face, eyelid margins, nasolabial folds, cheeks, eyebrows and forehead. Involvement of the outer ear occurs (otitis externa).

Pompholyx   Another variant of eczema affecting the hands and feet (Fig. 3.6), characterised by the eruption of itchy vesicles, especially on the lateral margins of the fingers and toes, as well as the palms and soles.

Varicose eczema   Occurs in patients with longstanding varicose veins. Eczematous patches affect the lower leg and may or may not be associated with other skin disorders caused by varicose veins; for example, venous ulcers that occur in the region of the medial maleolus, pigmentation and oedema.

Psoriasis   The lesions are well-defined, slightly raised and erythematous. In the chronic phase, silvery scales over the surface. The lesions vary in size from small (guttate) (Fig. 3.7) to large plaques (Fig. 3.8). These lesions are widely distributed over the body and may either resolve or persist as chronic psoriasis.

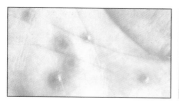

Fig. 3.6 Pompholyx: pruritic vesicles on the hand.

Fig. 3.7 Guttate (teardrop) psoriasis.

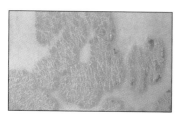

Fig. 3.8 Psoriatic plaque. Note the scaly, shiny surface and the sharp border.

Chronic psoriasis
The plaques of chronic psoriasis have a predeliction for the scalp, elbows, knees, perineum, umbilicus and submammary skin. The lesions are usually symmetrical. A characteristic feature of psoriasis is the development of new psoriatic lesions where the skin is traumatised (the Koebner phenomenon).

Pustular psoriasis
A variant, usually confined to the palms and soles, although some are occasionally more diffuse. The pustules, 2–5 mm in diameter, are yellow.

Psoriatic arthropathy
The distal interphalangeal joints are affected. Large joints may be affected, either singly or symmetrically. Rarely, patients may have sacroiliitis or even spinal ankylosis. The nails may be involved even in the absence of skin disease. The typical features include pinpoint pitting of the nail and onycholysis (lifting of the distal nail from the nail bed).

Pityriasis rosea
A common disorder in the younger patient. A single patch rash occurs days or even weeks before the more general eruption. This 'herald patch' may be confused with ringworm. The full blown rash affects the upper arms, trunk and upper thighs ('shirt and shorts' distribution). Pink papules evolve into 1–3 cm itchy oval macules that scale near the edge, giving a characteristic appearance. The rash resolve within 6 weeks.

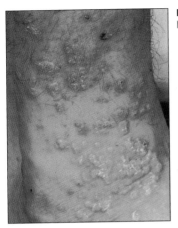

Fig. 3.9 Polygonal papules in lichen planus.

Lichen planus

Another itchy rash, diagnosed at the bedside by its typical appearance (Fig. 3.9).

The rash affects both the skin and mucous membranes. It has a predeliction for the volar (front) aspect of the forearm and wrists, the dorsal (back) surface of the hands, the shins, ankles and lower back region. The rash is symmetrical and characterised by small, shiny, purple or violaceous papules which have a polygonal rather than rounded outline. A network of white lines on the surface of the papules are termed Wickham's striae. Eruptions occur after trauma (Koebner phenomenon) and linear lesions are tell-tale signs occurring in scratched areas. The buccal mucous membrane is commonly involved.

SKIN INFECTIONS

Bacterial

IMPETIGO

Caused by β-haemolytic streptococci. The face is most commonly infected. Lesions start as a papular eruption around the mouth and nose that then evolves into a vesicular eruption and spreads locally. The lesion breaks down to leave a typical honey-coloured crust.

FURUNCLE (BOIL)

An infection of a hair follicle, caused by *Staphylococcus aureus*, that spreads locally into the surrounding tissue. A head of pus may be obvious at its apex. A local collection of furuncles is called a carbuncle. A stye (or hordeolum) is a small furuncle affecting an eyelash.

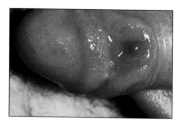

Fig. 3.10 Primary chancre in syphilis.

ERYSIPELAS AND CELLULITIS

Infection of the superficial skin layers by *Streptococcus pyogenes* is termed erysipelas, whereas an infection of the deeper skin layers is called cellulitis. Erysipelas is characterised by the abrupt onset of a well-demarcated slightly raised and tender erythematous rash. The patient is usually pyrexial and toxic. The margin of an area of cellulitis is less well defined than erysipelas.

SYPHILIS

In primary syphilis, a painless ulcer with an indurated edge (primary chancre) (Fig. 3.10) appears at the site of infection (usually on the genitalia). Approximately 2 months after the appearance of the chancre, the secondary rash appears: a pink macular rash on the trunk that becomes papular, affecting the genital skin, palms and soles. In the anal and groin regions, the moistness may cause erosions (codylomata accuminata). Raised oval patches occur in the mucous membrane of the mouth (snail-track ulcers). In the tertiary stage, granulomas form (gummas); these skin nodules are prone to degenerate and ulcerate.

Viral

WARTS

Warts usually occur on the fingers and hands as discrete papules with a typical irregular surface. Plantar warts occur on the pressure-bearing areas of the feet and are consequently flattened rather than raised.

MOLLUSCUM CONTAGIOSUM

A common infection caused by a member of the pox virus group. The lesions appear as flesh-coloured, dome-shaped papules varying in size from pinpoint to 1 cm in diameter. The most characteristic feature of the lesion is umbilication (a central depression of the surface).

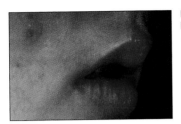

Fig. 3.11 'Fever blister' caused by herpes simplex.

HERPES SIMPLEX

Type 1 virus normally affects the mouth and lips (Fig. 3.11), whereas type 2 usually affects the genitals. The primary HSV infection presents with crops of painful superficial vesicles surrounded by an area of erythema. The vesicles erode superficially then crust and finally heal without scarring. After the primary infection, the virus lies dormant in the dorsal root nerve ganglion, with recurrences occurring predictably in the same area as the initial infection. Reactivation is heralded by a tingling sensation in the skin which is followed within 1–2 days by the eruption of a crop of vesicles.

HERPES ZOSTER (SHINGLES)

After an attack of chicken pox, the varicella-zoster virus lies dormant in a dorsal root or cranial nerve ganglion. Reactivation of the virus causes a localised eruption called shingles.

The patient complains of pain or discomfort in a localised area of skin and, within a few days, a crop of vesicles appear in a characteristic dermatomal distribution. Over 2–3 weeks, the vesicles evolve into pustules, scab, then heal. If the ophthalmic branch of the trigeminal nerve is involved, there may be serious damage to the cornea. This is associated with a typical distribution of the vesicles on the tip and side of the nose. Involvement of the geniculate ganglion of the facial nerve causes a facial palsy with involvement of the outer ear (Ramsay Hunt syndrome). The most debilitating long-term effect of shingles is chronic pain and hyperaesthesia in the affected dermatome.

Fungal

CANDIDA ALBICANS

Look for candidosis in the mouth; the oral infection is characterised by white or off-white plaques that can be scraped off, leaving a raw red base. Other manifestations include angular stomatitis, vulval and vaginal infections and involvement of contact surfaces (e.g. the natal cleft, inner thighs, scrotum and inframammary fold (intertrigo)).

PITYRIASIS VERSICOLOR (TINEA VERSICOLOR)

This common condition of young adults is caused by *Malassezia furfur* and presents as small pigmented or hypopigmented macules on the upper trunk and arms. In sunburnt areas, the lesions appear to be hypopigmented.

DERMATOPHYTES (TINEA)

Hair infection (tinea capitis) presents with localised patches of hair loss and skin inflammation. Skin infection (tinea corporis) affects the unhairy parts of the body. This presentation is often referred to as 'ringworm', because the lesion has an inflamed annular edge with a paler central area of healing. Athlete's foot (tinea pedis) appears as a scaling erythematous rash between the toes. A nail infection (tinea unguium) is often asymmetrical and affects the toenails more often than the fingernails. The nail becomes yellow and thick; there is onycholysis and the nail crumbles and breaks.

Infestations

PEDICULOSIS

Headlice infestation (pediculosis capitis) is common in children. The diagnosis is made by careful inspection of the hair for eggs (nits) which, unlike dandruff, cannot be shaken off the hair. Scratching may give rise to secondary inflammation and itching. Body lice infestation (pediculosis corporis) is rare. Infection of the pubic hair (pediculosis pubis) is caused by the crab louse and is usually sexually transmitted. The infestation causes intense pruritus and the nits (and lice) are seen with the naked eye.

SCABIES

The mite (*Sarcoptes scabei*) burrows into the skin, where the female lays her eggs. The burrows can be seen on inspection; look for these along the sides of the fingers, the webs and the wrist. The lesions may affect the elbows, axillae and genitalia. Scratching causes secondary excoriation and infection.

Blistering lesions

BULLOUS PEMPHIGOID

Occurs most commonly in elderly people. The lesions are itchy and appear as tense, mainly symmetrical blisters overlying and surrounded by an area of erythema. The blisters are initially small but enlarge to a considerable size over a few days (Fig. 3.12). The blisters appear mainly on the limbs, especially along the inner aspects of the thighs and arms. The blisters become haemorrhagic and degenerate, causing erosions that are susceptible to secondary infection.

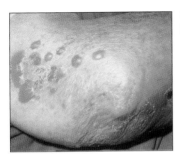

Fig. 3.12 Tense blisters of bullous pemphigoid.

PEMPHIGUS
Occurs most commonly in middle-aged Ashkenazi Jews. Lesions often start in the mouth or genital mucous membrane; however, patients usually present to the doctor once the skin is involved. Pemphigus is characterised by painful, flaccid blisters that rupture to reveal a raw base that heals slowly. The skin adjacent to the bullous lesion slides over the underlying dermis (Nikolsky's sign). The umbilicus, trunk, intertrigenous areas and scalp are most commonly affected.

DERMATITIS HERPETIFORMIS
Characterised by strikingly symmetrical groups of intensely itchy vesicles which most commonly erupt on the elbows, below the knees, buttocks, back and scalp. Scratching causes local excoriation. Healing leaves tell-tale areas of hyperpigmentation. The disorder is almost always associated with gluten-sensitive enteropathy (coeliac disease).

NAEVI
The junctional naevus is distinguished as a flat or slightly raised smooth lesion which has a uniform colour and varies in size up to about 1 cm. A compound naevus is a raised, rounded, pigmented papular lesion from which hairs may project. Dermal naevi are raised, flesh-coloured, dome-shaped lesions with a wrinkled surface, occurring most commonly on the face.

CAFÉ AU LAIT PATCHES
Are flat, coffee-coloured patches, usually centimetres in size, which may occur as a benign blemish or a marker of neurofibromatosis. The presence of five or more of these patches is a sure sign of the disorder. Neurofibromas appear as soft, sessile, pedunculated lesions or discrete subcutaneuous nodules.

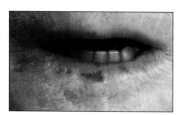

Fig. 3.13 Squamous cancer of the lip.

Tumours

SQUAMOUS CELL CARCINOMA
Presents as an ulcer or nodule with a firm indurated margin; the ulcer margin is often everted (Fig. 3.13). The cancer usually occurs in sun-exposed areas.

BASAL CELL CARCINOMA
Most commonly affects the face and, like squamous carcinoma, sun-exposure is an important predisposing factor. The 'rodent' ulcer starts as a small painless papule which ulcerates. The ulcer margin is well-defined and rolled at the edges. The tumour bleeds and scabs.

MALIGNANT MELANOMA
The tumour is usually pigmented and presents either as a nodule or a spreading area of pigmentation. Consider the diagnosis if a pigmented lesion is nodular, grows, darkens in colour, changes shape or bleeds. The back is a common site in men, whereas in women the legs are the most common site.

KAPOSI'S SARCOMA
Once restricted to equatorial black Africans and elderly Ashkenazi Jews. Immunosuppression is an important predisposing factor and the sarcoma occurs in transplant recipients on immunosuppressive drugs and is particularly associated with AIDS. The Kaposi's lesion is characterised by red–blue nodules, especially affecting the lower legs but also involving the hands.

NAIL DISORDERS

Asymmetrical splinter-like lesions (splinter haemorrhages) may indicate microemboli from infected heart valves (subacute bacterial endocarditis) or vasculitis. Pitting of the nail occurs in psoriasis and may even occur in the absence of the typical skin rash. Premature

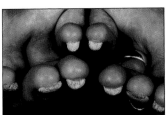

Fig. 3.14   Onycholysis caused by hyperkeratotic psoriasis beneath the nail.

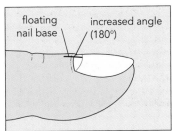

Fig. 3.15   Clubbing. The angle is increased and filled in and the nail base has a spongy consistency.

lifting of the distal nail is called onycholysis (Fig. 3.14). This occurs in many nail disorders and is also associated with hyperthyroidism (Plummer's nails). White nails with loss of the lunule (leukonychia) is typical of hypoalbuminaemia and severe chronic ill-health.

Acute severe illness may be associated with the later appearance of transverse depressions in the nail (Beau's lines) which grow out with normal nail growth on recovery. Infection of the skin adjacent to the nail is called paronychia and is characterised by pain, swelling, redness and tenderness of the skin at its interface with the nail. Spooning of the nail (koilonychia) occurs in iron deficiency.

Always examine the lateral outline of the nails and fingertip to check for clubbing. The normal angle between the fingernail and nail base is 160° (Fig. 3.15) and the base is firm to palpation. In early clubbing, the angle increases and if you press the nail base the nail appears to 'float'. In severe clubbing, such as occurs with lung cancer, the fingers may have a drumstick appearance and may be associated with wrist pain and tenderness due to periostitis (hypertrophic pulmonary osteoarthropathy).

SKIN MANIFESTATIONS OF SYSTEMIC DISEASE

Many systemic disorders involve the skin and careful examination of the skin often helps in diagnosis.

Symptoms and signs
Skin manifestations of systemic disease

Disease	Skin findings
Sarcoidosis	Erythema nodosum, lupus pernio, nodules in scars
Systemic lupus erythematosus	Facial 'butterfly' rash (malar erythema over cheeks and bridging nose); occurs in 50% of patients on exposure to UV rays. Also alopoecia areata and discoid lupus
Scleroderma	Thickened tight skin (especially fingers), skin telangiectasia, calcified skin nodules
Hyperlipidaemia	Xanthelasmata of eyelids, xanthomas of elbows, knuckles, buttock, soles and palms, and Achilles tendon
Diabetes mellitus	Necrobiosis lipoidica – symmetrical plaques on shins with atrophic, yellow appearance and waxy feel; cutaneous candida, ulcers on feet
Hyperthyroidism	Pretibial myxoedema – thickened skin on front of shin, clubbing
Cushing's syndrome	Purple striae, thin skin, easy bruising
Ulcerative colitis/ Crohn's disease	Pyoderma gangrenosum – large ulcer
Deramtomyositis	Oedema and mauve discoloration of eyelid, erythema of the knuckles and other bony parts such as elbow and shoulder tip; photosensitive 'butterfly rash' on face
Cancer	Acanthosis nigricans – brown, velvet-like thickening of skin in axilla and groin; tylosis – thickening of palms/soles; ichthyosis – fish-skin appearance

 Examination of elderly people
Skin changes in elderly people

- Skin becomes increasingly wrinkled with loss of elastic tissue and collagen
- Skin becomes fragile and even minor trauma can cause wounding and secondary infection
- Loss of spring makes it more difficult to use tissue turgor as a sign for assessing hydration
- Capillary fragility results in easy intradermal bleeding (senile purpura and ecchymosis)

Examination of elderly people
Skin changes in elderly people – *(cont'd)*

- Warty pigmented lesions (senile keratosis) may become widespread and disfigure skin
- Sunburnt area increasingly predisposed to malignant change in the elderly (squamous and basal cell carcinomas)
- Pressure sores (decubitus ulcers) are a particularly serious complication of immobility; predisposing factors include capillary occlusion, friction and secondary infection
- Pressure sores most commonly develop over bony prominences, especially the heels and sacrum

 Review
Skin examination

- Always expose the patient to allow examination of the whole skin organ
- Ensure good illumination (preferably natural light)
- Measure dimensions of skin lesions (especially helpful when assessing progression and regression)
- Attempt to transilluminate larger swellings (fluid-filled)
- Assess skin colour and variations
- Describe the primary morphology of a localised skin lesion
  - macule
  - patch
  - papule
  - plaque
  - wheal
  - vesicle
  - nodule
  - petechia or ecchymosis
  - bulla
  - telangiectasia, spider naevus
- Describe the secondary characteristics
  - superficial erosion
  - ulceration
  - crusting
  - scaling
  - fissuring
  - lichenification
  - atrophy
  - excoriation
  - scarring or keloid
- Describe the distribution of a more widespread rash or colour change
- Assess the temperature of the affected area
- Perform a general examination, looking for evidence of systemic disease

4.
Ear, Nose and Throat

SYMPTOMS OF MOUTH AND THROAT DISORDERS

Patients with disorders arising in the mouth or throat usually complain of pain, a sensation of a lump in the throat, a hoarse voice, difficulty in breathing (upper airway obstruction), difficulty in swallowing (dysphagia), pain on swallowing (odynophagia), a lump in the neck and halitosis (bad breath).

Sore throat or mouth

Pain may arise from the teeth or from the buccal and lingual surfaces. The oral mucosa may be diffusely inflamed in vitamin-deficiency states, in fungal infections of the oral cavity ('thrush' or candidiasis) or after radiotherapy for malignant disease. Diffuse fungal infection should alert you to the possibility of AIDS, although it may also occur after broad-spectrum antibiotic therapy or in any state of immune deficiency (e.g. leukaemia, lymphoma). Pain arising more posteriorly may be due to tonsillitis or pharyngitis which can be seen but may also be due to disease of the hypo- and laryngopharynx.

Specific lesions of the oral and buccal mucosa are inflammatory (most commonly aphthous ulcers), traumatic or due to a localised malignancy.

Questions to ask
Sore mouth or throat

- How long have you had the pain?
- Does the pain change in severity?
- What aggravates and what relieves the pain?
- Is the pain local or diffuse?
- What other illnesses do you have?
- Are you taking any medications; if so, what type?
- How much do you smoke a day?
- How much alcohol do you consume in a week?

Lump in the throat

Previously known as globus hystericus this is now more appropriately called globus pharyngeus or the globus syndrome. It is described as a sensation of 'something' or a 'lump' in the throat.

Hoarse voice

The majority of patients with a hoarse voice have an inflammatory disorder of the larynx (laryngitis). Any patient with hoarseness that has not resolved after 3 weeks should have the larynx visualised.

The history will often give the examiner a good idea of the diagnosis. Any alteration in the smooth lining of the true vocal cords (vocal folds) will give rise to hoarseness. If one of the vocal folds is paralysed or if there is inadequate apposition of the vocal folds, a more 'breathy' quality of the voice is noted and is more accurately called dysphonia. A preceding upper respiratory tract infection will usually point to a diagnosis of laryngitis, as may excessive voice abuse (traumatic laryngitis). Excessive smoking, alcohol (especially spirits) and poor periodontal and dental hygiene should alert you to the possibility of a malignancy.

Obstructed airway

Snoring is caused by an obstructed airway. The obstruction may be nasal, postnasal (e.g. enlarged adenoid), oropharyngeal (e.g. tonsils, lax palate and faucial pillars) or laryngeal (e.g. congenital abnormalities in children). If snoring is severe it may be associated with apnoeic episodes during sleep.

Difficulty in swallowing

For a discussion of difficulty in swallowing (dysphagia) see Chapter 7.

Pain on swallowing

Painful swallowing is called odynophagia. Swallowing is usually painful in the presence of inflammation in the hypopharynx or oesophagus (e.g. candidiasis). Carcinoma of the piriform fossa or posterior one-third of the tongue may present with odynophagia.

Lump in the neck

Most neck lumps are due to enlarged lymph nodes, in which case questioning is directed to a potential source of origin (Fig. 4.1). Enlarged lymph nodes in the neck may arise from sources in the head

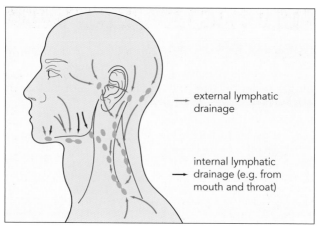

Fig. 4.1 Lymphatic drainage of the head and neck.

> ? Questions to ask
> **Lump in the neck**
>
> - How long has it been present?
> - Has the lump changed in size?
> - Is the lump painful?
> - Do you sweat at night?
> - Have you lost weight recently?
> - Do you have thyroid problems?
> - Do you have a cough?
> - Is there anything abnormal about your mouth or throat?
> - Are you generally well?

and neck. Thyroid swellings would require a history of symptoms of hyperthyroidism or hypothyroidism.

Halitosis

The most common cause of halitosis is probably poor dental and oral hygiene. Paranasal sinus infection with a purulent postnasal discharge may lead to halitosis, as may tonsillar crypts. Infection of the oral cavity, the gums in particular (gingivitis), may give rise to foul-smelling breath.

SYMPTOMS OF NASAL DISORDERS

Blocked nose

Mechanical abnormalities (e.g. a deviated septum or enlarged turbinates or nasal polyps) will usually cause constant obstruction; seasonal allergic rhinitis are usually intermittent.

Questions to ask
Blocked nose

- Is the nose blocked constantly or only some of the time (day or night)?
- Does it vary with the seasons?
- Is there any associated nasal discharge?
- Are both nostrils affected or only one?
- What aggravates and what relieves the condition?
- Do you use nose drops?
- Do you sniff glue or illicit substances (e.g. cocaine)?
- Have you had previous nose surgery?
- Do you suffer from asthma?

Runny nose (rhinorrhoea)

Ascertain whether there is associated nasal obstruction and whether the discharge is constant or intermittent (as in seasonal rhinitis). The discharge may be watery or mucoid, purulent in the presence of infection or a foreign body (children or mentally handicapped adults) and blood stained in the presence of a tumour. If rhinorrhoea is associated with an itchy nose, sneezing and itchy eyes, a diagnosis of allergic rhinitis can easily be made.

Bleeding nose (epistaxis)

A history of a bleeding disorder is relevant, as is a history of previous nasal surgery: septal perforations often crust and bleed. Nose bleeds may be caused by excessive nasal picking.

'Nonsmelling' nose

Patients may complain of a diminished sense of smell (hyposmia) or no sense of smell (anosmia). There may be a history of head injury. Some patients may report a loss of the sense of smell after an upper respiratory tract infection. Patients with nasal polyps or mucosal oedema in allergic rhinitis will also complain of anosmia. In many patients the cause is unknown.

SYMPTOMS OR EAR DISORDERS

Painful ear (otolgia)

Pain in the ear arises from the ear itself or is referred from several other anatomical sites. Disorders of the nose and sinuses, nasopharynx, teeth, jaws, temporomandibular joints, salivary glands and ducts, oropharynx, laryngopharynx and hypopharynx, tongue and cervical spine may all give rise to earache.

 Questions to ask
Otalgia

- Where does it hurt?
- Does the pain spread?
- What exacerbates the pain?
- Is there a discharge?
- Have you ever had an ear operation or your ears syringed?
- Do you use cotton buds?
- Have you hurt your ear recently?
- Have you been swimming or on an aeroplane recently?
- Is your hearing ability affected?

Discharging ear (otorrhoea)

Discharge may contain mucus or pus, and may be bloodstained. Earache and discharge often coexist.

Hearing loss or deafness

The age of onset of the hearing loss is important, as is the suddenness of its onset.

'Noisy' ear (tinnitus)

Tinnitus usually presents as buzzing, whistling, hissing, ringing or pulsating. Tinnitus is usually associated with a degree of hearing loss, yet it may occur without any hearing loss. The cause and site of origin of the noise in subjective tinnitus is usually unknown.

Deformed ear

Congenital ear deformities include complete or partial absence of the pinna (anotia or microtia). This may be associated with middle and inner ear abnormalities.

Patients may also complain about the size or shape of their ears, particularly if the ears protrude. This condition can be corrected surgically.

Injury to the ear

Trauma may have occurred in the external meatus, usually self-inflicted (e.g. with cotton buds, hairgrips or pencils). Blunt trauma in the form of a blow to the side of the head or in diffuse head injury may rupture the tympanic membrane, dislocate the ossicles and cause damage to the inner ear.

Vertigo

Vertigo is an hallucination of movement. Feelings of 'light headedness', 'about to black out or faint', do not constitute true vertigo.

In general, central causes of vertigo are more constant and are progressive, whereas vestibular causes tend to be intermittent and paroxysmal and are not usually progressive.

Facial pain

The source may be relatively obvious (e.g. the patient may say 'I have toothache') or the pain may be referred from a distant site (e.g. the patient with tonsillitis who complains of earache).

Facial nerve palsy

A history of ear disease is particularly relevant because the facial nerve makes a considerable journey through the temporal bone, crossing the medial wall of the middle ear, the mastoid, before making its exit at the stylomastoid foramen. Questions relating to the function of branches of the facial nerve, such as dry eyes (if the greater superficial petrosal nerve is involved) or altered taste (if the chorda tympani is involved) can give you an idea of the level of nerve disruption.

EXAMINATION OF THE MOUTH AND THROAT

Examine the lips for telangiectasia, ulcers, pigmentation and cracks. Inspect the buccal mucosa, gums and teeth. If the patient wears dentures, these should be removed. Note the state of periodontal

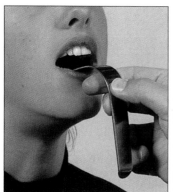

Fig. 4.2 Examining the mouth using a tongue depressor.

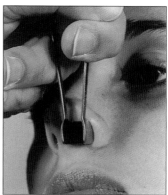

Fig. 4.3 Anterior rhinoscopy using a Thudicum speculum.

hygiene and any evidence of gingivitis (inflammation of the gums). Inspect the hard palate for evidence of a cleft palate or a repaired cleft and for telangiectasia.

Next, ask the patient to protrude the tongue. Ask the patient to touch the palate with the tongue to allow you to see the floor of the mouth with the submandibular ducts opening on either side of the frenulum. Look for ulcers, nodules, furring and leukoplakia (white patches) on the tongue. Ask the patient to say 'aaah'. This will allow you to see the tonsils, the posterior pharyngeal wall and the movement of the soft palate. You may require a tongue depressor to obtain an adequate view of the posterior aspects of the oral cavity and oropharynx (Fig. 4.2).

Finally, put on a glove and feel any suspicious areas within the mouth.

EXAMINATION OF THE NOSE

Examine the nasal vestibule. In children, the cartilages of the nasal tip are soft and a good view of the nasal vestibule, anterior end of the septum and anterior ends of the inferior turbinates can be obtained by simply elevating the tip of the nose. In adults, the cartilages are firmer and the use of a Thudicum speculum is usually necessary to obtain a similar view (Fig. 4.3).

Ask the patient to breath out nasally and observe the resultant moisture on a silver tongue depressor or mirror positioned at the anterior nares. The inspiratory flow can be assessed crudely by

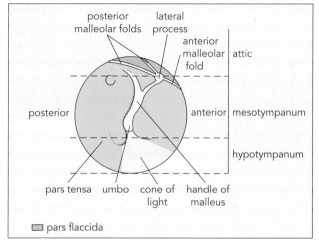

Fig. 4.4 Anatomy of normal tympanic membrane.

occluding the undersurface of one nasal cavity at a time and asking the patient to sniff. To assess the sense of smell ask the patient to identify the smells from simple smell bottles, although this is not particularly reliable.

EXAMINATION OF THE EAR

Examine the pinna, note its shape, size and any deformity. Feel for preauricular, postauricular and infra-auricular lymph nodes, the result of external ear disease.

Observe the meatus. An auroscope with a puffer attached is then used to examine the deep meatus and tympanic membrane. Apply gentle traction on the ear to straighten the external ear canal and gently insert the auroscope.

Introduce the auroscope and look at the canal wall skin for otitis externa and exostoses. Severe otitis external or a boil (furuncle) of the external meatus may totally occlude the meatus. Gently remove the wax by using a ring probe, a wax hook or a suction apparatus. If the wax is very hard, it may be possible to use a wax softener (e.g. olive oil or sodium bicarbonate ear drops) for a few days before attempting its removal.

The tympanic membrane is inspected next. All anatomical features of the drum should be actively sought and noted (Fig. 4.4). Note the presence of absence of any perforation. An accumulation of white epithelial debris indicates the presence of cholesteatoma.

The puffer is used next. This is valuable in assessing mobility of the tympanic membrane. As the puffer is squeezed, the drum should be seen to move medially then laterally. An immobile tympanic membrane indicates there is an inadequate seal with escape of air, a tympanic membrane perforation is present or there is an effusion in the middle ear.

Hearing should be assessed using tuning forks. It is also possible to perform a crude assessment of the hearing by whispering at various distances.

Questions to ask
Hearing loss

- How long have you noticed a hearing loss?
- Is it partial or complete?
- Are both the ears affected or just one?
- Is there a family history of hearing problems?
- Have you had an injury or surgery to your ears?
- Have you had any serious illnesses such as tuberculosis or septicaemia (ototoxic drugs)?
- Have you been exposed to loud noise for any length of time?
- Is there associated vertigo?

Differential diagnosis
Hearing loss

Infants	Congenital
	Secretory otitis media ('glue ear')
Toddlers and young children	'Glue ear'
	Congenital
	Postinfective (measles, mumps, meningitis)
Teenagers and adolescents	Congenital
	Malingering
	Postinfective
	Noise induced (often temporary in this age group)
20–40 years old	Otosclerosis
	Postinfective
	Noise induced
	Acoustic neuroma
	Ménière's disease

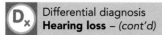

Dx Differential diagnosis
Hearing loss – *(cont'd)*

40–60 years old	Otosclerosis
	Noise induced
	Early presbycusis
	Acoustic neuroma
	Ménière's disease
Above 60 years old	Presbycusis
	Noise induced
	Acoustic neuroma

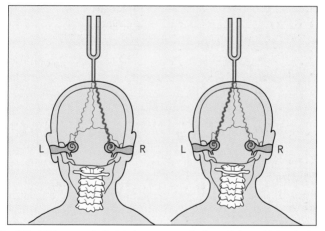

Fig. 4.5 Weber test. Left-sided perceptive deafness (left) and left-sided conductive hearing loss (right).

The Weber test

The Weber test is first performed by putting the vibrating tuning fork (Fig. 4.5) on the midline of the patient's skull. Ask the patient where the vibration is heard. If the hearing is normal in both ears or the hearing loss is symmetrical, the vibration will be heard in the middle or equally in both ears. The vibration is heard in only one ear if that particular ear has a conductive hearing loss.

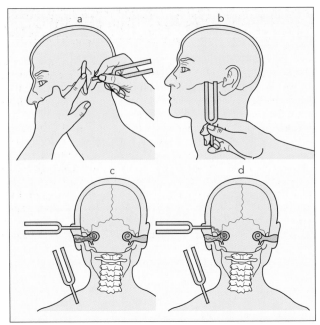

Fig. 4.6 Rinne test. Comparison of (a) bone conduction and (b) air conduction. (c) Normal: air conduction better than bone conduction. (d) Conductive hearing loss: bone conduction better than air conduction.

The Rinne test

The Rinne test (Fig. 4.6) should be performed in conjunction with the Weber test. The base of the vibrating tuning fork is placed against the patient's mastoid process. When the patient can no longer hear the vibration, the turning fork is placed next to the ear on that side. If the sound is now heard, the Rinne test is positive. This implies that air conduction is better than bone conduction and that there is no significant conductive hearing loss. The test is then repeated for the opposite ear. If the tuning fork is heard better over the mastoid process, then the Rinne test is negative; that is, bone conduction is better than air conduction.

Formal audiometric testing

In pure tone and speech audiometry, the patient is asked to respond to different pure tones and speech and the response is recorded. Objective testing aims to eliminate subjectivity and malingering.

EXAMINATION OF THE NECK AND TEMPOROMANDIBULAR JOINTS

The neck and temporomandibular joints should be examined next. The temporomandibular joints are palpated just anterior to the tragus of the ear. The patient is asked to open the mouth as the joint is palpated. Feel for clicking or crepitus over the joint and ask the patient if the joint is painful when palpated.

The neck should be palpated after looking at its shape and contours. Palpate the neck in a systematic pattern (e.g. submental triangle, submandibular regions, posterior and anterior triangles). When the patient swallows, locate and assess the thyroid gland and any thyroid or midline neck swellings. The thyroid gland and thyroglossal duct remnants move upwards on swallowing. Feel and auscultate the carotid arteries for any bruits. Active and passive movements of flexion, extension, rotation and lateral flexion should be performed to assess limitation of movement, induction of pain, or paraesthesiae in the upper limbs.

5.
Respiratory System

Important for the examiner is the arrangement of the lobes of the lungs (Fig. 5.1). It will be seen that both lungs are divided into two and the right lung is divided again to form the middle lobe. The corresponding area on the left is the lingula, a division of the upper lobe. Examination of the front of the chest is largely that of the upper lobes, examination of the back the lower lobes.

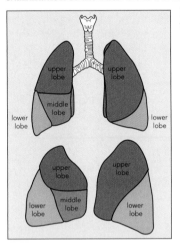

Fig. 5.1 Lobes of the lung: anterior view (upper) and lateral view (lower).

SYMPTOMS OF RESPIRATORY DISEASE

Dyspnoea

 Questions to ask
Dyspnoea

- Is the breathlessness recent or has it been present for sometime?
- Is it constant or does it come and go?
- What can't you do because of the breathlessness?
- What makes the breathing worse?
- Does anything make it better?

CAUSES OF BREATHLESSNESS

 Differential diagnosis
Some causes of breathlessness

Control and movement of the chest wall and pleura
- Hyperventilation syndrome
- Hypothalamic lesions
- Neuromuscular disease
- Kyphoscoliosis
- Akylosing spondylitis
- Pleural effusion and thickening
- Bilateral diaphragm paralysis

Diseases of the lungs
- Airways disease
  - chronic bronchitis and emphysema
  - asthma
  - bronchiectasis
  - cystic fibrosis
- Parenchymal disease
  - pneumonia
  - cryptogenic fibrosing alveolitis
  - extrinsic allergic alveolitis
  - primary and secondary tumour
  - sarcoidosis
  - pneumothorax
  - pulmonary oedema
- Reduced blood supply
  - pulmonary embolism
  - anaemia

DURATION OF DYSPNOEA

 Differential diagnosis
Duration of breathlessness

Immediate (minutes)
- Pulmonary embolism
- Pneumothorax
- Pulmonary oedema
- Asthma

Differential diagnosis
Duration of breathlessness – *(cont'd)*

Short (hours to days)
- Pulmonary oedema
- Pneumonia
- Asthma
- Pleural effusion
- Anaemia

Long (weeks to years)
- Chronic airflow limitation
- Cryptogenic fibrosing alveolitis
- Extrinsic allergic alveolitis
- Anaemia

ASTHMA

Asthma due solely to emotional causes probably does not exist; nonetheless, most patients who have asthma are worse if emotionally upset. Nocturnal asthma is very common.

 Questions to ask
Asthma

- Does anything make any difference to the asthma?
- What happens if you are worried or upset?
- Does your chest wake you at night?
- Does cigarette smoke make any difference?
- Do household sprays affect you?
- Have you lost time from work/school?
- What happens when sweeping or dusting the house?
- Does exposure to cats or dogs make any difference?

SEVERITY OF DYSPNOEA

Severity can be assessed by rating scales, although it is much better to use some functional measure. Ask patients in what way their breathlessness restricts their activities: can they go upstairs, go shopping, wash the car or do the garden? If they are troubled with stairs, how many flights can they manage? It is important to be certain that any restriction is caused by breathlessness and not some other disability (e.g. an arthritic hip or angina).

ORTHOPNOEA AND PAROXYSMAL NOCTURNAL DYSPNOEA

Orthopnoea is defined as breathlessness lying flat but relieved by sitting up. It is common in patients with severe fixed airways obstruction.

Paroxysmal nocturnal dyspnoea is a feature of pulmonary oedema from left ventricular failure. However, many asthmatics develop bronchoconstriction in the night and wake with wheeze and breathlessness very similar to the symptoms of left ventricular failure.

THE HYPERVENTILATION SYNDROME

Symptoms and signs
Features suggestive of the hyperventilation syndrome

- Breathlessness at rest
- Breathlessness as severe with mild exertion as with greater exertion
- Marked variability in breathlessness
- More difficulty breathing in than out
- Paraesthesiae of the fingers
- Numbness around the mouth
- 'Lightheadedness'
- Feelings of impending collapse or remoteness from surroundings
- Chest wall pain

Cough

Cough may be the only symptom in asthma, particularly childhood asthma. In children, cough occurring regularly after exercise or at night is virtually diagnostic of asthma.

Laryngitis will cause both cough and a hoarse voice. Cough from tracheitis is usually dry and painful. Cough from further down the airways is often associated with sputum production (bronchitis, bronchiectasis or pneumonia). Other possibilities are carcinoma, lung fibrosis and increased bronchial responsiveness. An uncommon cause of cough and often overlooked is aspiration into the lungs from gastro-oesophageal reflux or a pharyngeal pouch. Cough will then follow meals or lying down. Prolonged coughing bouts can cause both unconsciousness from reduction of venous return to the brain (cough syncope) and also vomiting.

Sputum

Questions on frequency are most useful in the diagnosis of chronic bronchitis, an epidemiological definition of this is 'sputum production on most days for 3 consecutive months for 2 successive years'. The diagnosis of bronchiectasis is made on a story of daily sputum production stretching back to childhood.

Sticky 'rusty' sputum is characteristic of lobar pneumonia, and frothy sputum with streaks of blood is seen in pulmonary oedema.

Questions to ask
Sputum

- What colour is the phlegm?
- How often do you bring it up?
- How much do you bring up?
- Do you have trouble getting it up?

Symptoms and signs
Sputum

White or grey
- Smoking
- Simple chronic bronchitis
- Asthma

Yellow or green
- Acute bronchitis
- Acute on chronic bronchitis
- Asthma
- Bronchiectasis
- Cystic fibrosis

Frothy, blood-streaked
- Pulmonary oedema

Haemoptysis

The blood in haemoptysis is usually bright red at first, then followed by progressively smaller and darker amounts.

All haemoptysis is potentially serious, although the most important is carcinoma of the bronchus. Repeated small haemoptysis every few days over a period of some weeks in a middle-aged smoker is virtually diagnostic of bronchial carcinoma.

Differential diagnosis
Haemoptysis

Common
- Infection including bronchiectasis
- Bronchial carcinoma
- Tuberculosis
- Pulmonary embolism and infarction
- No cause found

Uncommon
- Mitral stenosis and left ventricular failure
- Bronchial adenoma
- Idiopathic pulmonary haemosiderosis
- Anticoagulation and blood dyscrasias

Risk factors
Pulmonary embolism

- Previous DVT or PE
- Surgery
- Immobility, especially stroke and heart failure
- Malignancy
- Pregnancy
- Leg trauma
- Haematological abnormalities

Pain

The lungs and the visceral pleura are devoid of pain fibres, whereas the parietal pleura, chest wall and mediastinal structures are not. The characteristic 'pleuritic pain' is sharp, stabbing, worse on deep breathing and coughing and arises from either pleural inflammation or chest wall lesions. Inflammation of the pleura occurs chiefly in pneumonia and pulmonary infarction from pulmonary emboli. Pneumothorax can produce acute transient pleuritic pain.

Most pains from the chest wall are caused by localised muscle strain or rib fractures (persistent cough can cause the latter). These pains are often worse on twisting or turning or rolling over in bed. Bornholm disease is thought to be a viral infection of the intercostal muscles and produces very severe pain. True pleuritic pain is often accompanied by a pleural rub. A particular type of chest wall pain is caused by swelling of one or more of the upper costal cartilages (Tietze's syndrome). Herpes zoster may cause pain in a root distribution round the chest.

Wheeze and stridor

WHEEZE
Wheeze occurs in both inspiration and expiration but is always louder in the latter. It implies airway narrowing and is common in asthma and chronic obstructive bronchitis. In asthma, the wheeze is episodic and clearly associated with shortness of breath, fulfilling the definition of 'variable wheezy breathlessness'.

STRIDOR
Stridor is a harsh inspiratory and expiratory noise which can be imitated by adducting the vocal cords and breathing in and out.

Other important points in the history

OTHER BODY SYSTEMS
Lung disease can affect the right side of the heart (cor pulmonale). An early manifestation is peripheral oedema (ankle swelling). Disease of the left heart causes pulmonary oedema (orthopnoea, paroxysmal nocturnal dyspnoea, cough and frothy sputum). Systems that affect the lungs include rheumatoid arthritis, other connective tissue disease (scleroderma and dermatomyositis), immune deficiency syndromes (including AIDS) and renal failure. A variety of neuromuscular diseases and skeletal problems affect the mechanics of breathing.

Weight loss is an important manifestation of lung carcinoma. Less well known is chronic airflow limitation, caused presumably by the increased respiratory effort impairing appetite and diverting calories to the respiratory muscles. Chronic infection, particularly tuberculosis, causes weight loss.

Fever generally implies infection, particularly pneumonia or tuberculosis. If pulmonary embolism is suspected, pain or swelling in the legs suggests a deep venous thrombosis.

SLEEP
In the sleep apnoea syndrome, patients are aroused repeatedly in the night from obstruction of the upper airways.

Previous disease

A history of tuberculosis may explain abnormal shadowing on a chest radiograph. Bronchial damage from tuberculosis can lead to bronchiectasis.

Symptoms and signs
Clinical features suggesting the sleep apnoea syndrome

- Excessive daytime somnolence
- Intellectual deterioration and irritability
- Early morning headaches
- Snoring
- Restless nights
- Social deterioration (e.g. job, marriage, driving difficulties)

A history of wheeze in childhood suggests asthma. Whooping cough or pneumonia in childhood may lead to bronchiectasis.

Social history

SMOKING
Smoking is, for practical purposes, the cause of chronic bronchitis and carcinoma of the bronchus.

Ask nonsmokers 'have you smoked in the past?'. The risk of disease increases with the amount smoked. Cigarettes are the most dangerous; pipes and cigars are not free of risk. Risk declines steadily when smoking stops; it takes 10–20 years for the risk of lung cancer to equal that of lifelong nonsmokers.

Inhalation of another person's smoke at home or at work is increasingly recognised as a factor in lung disease.

Risk factors
Lung cancer

- Smoking
- Atmospheric pollution
- Asbestos exposure
- Radon exposure (natural and occupational)
- Work in gas and coal industry

PETS AND HOBBIES
For many asthmatics, cats and dogs are common sources of allergen.

Exposure to racing pigeons, budgerigars, parrots and other caged birds can cause extrinsic allergic alveolitis. Acute symptoms are usually seen in pigeon fanciers who, a few hours after cleaning out their birds, develop cough, breathlessness and 'flu-like' symptoms. Chronic symptoms are seen in budgerigar owners.

Parrots and related species transmit the infectious agent of psittacosis, a cause of pneumonia.

OCCUPATION

 Risk factors
Some occupational causes of lung disease

Occupation	Agent	Disease
Mining	Coal dust	Pneumoconiosis
Quarrying	Silica dust	Silicosis
Foundry work	Silica dust	Silicosis
Asbestos	Asbestos fibres	Asbestosis
(Mining, heating,		Mesothelioma
building,		Lung cancer
demolition)		
Farming	Actinomycetes	Alveolitis
Paint spraying	Isocyanates	Asthma
Plastics manufacture	Isocyanates	Asthma
Soldering	Colophony	Asthma

Family history

The most common lung disease with a genetic basis is asthma. Other diseases that run in the family include cystic fibrosis and α_1-antitrypsin deficiency, a rare cause of emphysema.

Drug history

Aspirin and sometimes other nonsteroidal anti-inflammatory drugs and β-adrenergic receptor blockers can make asthma worse, and angiotensin-converting enzyme inhibitors cause chronic dry cough.

GENERAL EXAMINATION

First impressions

How breathless does the patient appear? Can the patient carry on a conversation with you or does he or she break up sentences? How breathless is the patient when getting undressed? Is there stridor or wheeze? Is there cough? Is there evidence of weight loss suggesting carcinoma? Does the patient have to sit up to breathe?

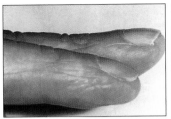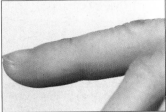

Fig. 5.2 Mild clubbing. The nail on the left shows obliteration of the angle at the nail fold compared with a normal nail on the right.

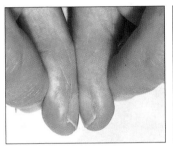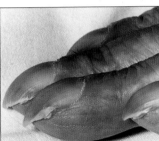

Fig. 5.3 Clubbing, showing how the diamond-shaped area is obliterated.

Fig. 5.4 Gross clubbing.

CLUBBING

The earliest stage is some softening of the nail bed, which can be detected by rocking the nail from side to side on the nail bed. Next, the soft tissue of the nail bed fills in the normal obtuse angle between the nail and the nail bed. The area becomes flat, even convex in clubbing (Fig. 5.2). This is seen best by viewing the nail from the side against a white background, say the bedsheets. When normal nails are placed 'back to back' there is usually a diamond-shaped area between them. This is obliterated early in clubbing (Fig. 5.3). In final stage, the whole tip of the finger becomes rounded (a club) (Fig. 5.4).

CYANOSIS

Cyanosis, a bluish tinge to the skin and mucous membranes, is seen when there is an increased amount of reduced haemoglobin in the blood. It becomes visible when there is approximately 5 g/dl or more of reduced haemoglobin, corresponding to a saturation of approximately 85%. Severe anaemia and cyanosis cannot coexist, otherwise most of the haemoglobin would be reduced. Conversely, in polycythaemia, in which there is an increase in red cell mass, there may be

Differential diagnosis
Some common causes of clubbing

Pulmonary
- Bronchial carcinoma
- Chronic pulmonary sepsis
  - empyema
  - lung abscess
  - bronchiectasis
  - cystic fibrosis
- Cryptogenic fibrosing alveolitis
- Asbestosis

Cardiac
- Congenital cyanotic heart disease
- Bacterial endocarditis

Other
- Idiopathic/familial
- Cirrhosis
- Ulcerative colitis
- Coeliac disease
- Crohn's disease

enough reduced haemoglobin to produce cyanosis, even though there is enough oxygenated haemoglobin to maintain a normal oxygen-carrying capacity.

CENTRAL CYANOSIS
The best place to look is the mucous membranes of the lips and tongue. The most common causes are severe airflow limitation, left ventricular failure and pulmonary fibrosis.

PERIPHERAL CYANOSIS
The peripheries, the fingers and the toes, are blue with normal mucous membranes. The usual cause is reduced circulation to the limbs, as seen in cold weather, Raynaud's phenomenon or peripheral vascular disease.

Cyanosis can rarely be caused by the abnormal pigments methaemo-globin and sulphaemoglobin. Arterial oxygen tension is normal.

TREMORS AND CARBON DIOXIDE RETENTION
Carbon dioxide retention is seen in severe chronic airflow limitation. Clinically, it can be suspected by a flapping tremor (indistinguishable from that associated with hepatic failure), vasodilatation manifested by warm peripheries, bounding pulses, papilloedema and headache.

PULSE AND BLOOD PRESSURE

Pulsus paradoxus is a drop in blood pressure on inspiration. A minor degree occurs normally. Major degrees occur in pericardial effusion and constrictive pericarditis but also in severe asthma.

JUGULAR VENOUS PULSE AND COR PULMONALE

The jugular venous pulse may be raised in cor pulmonale (right-sided heart failure due to lung disease). Other signs are peripheral oedema, hepatomegaly and a left parasternal heave, indicating right ventricular hypertrophy. In severe cases, functional tricuspid regurgitation will lead to a pulsatile liver, large V waves in the jugular venous pulse and a systolic murmur in tricuspid regurgitation.

LYMPHADENOPATHY

Lymphatics from the lungs drain centrally to the hilum, then up the paratracheal chain to the supraclavicular (scalene) or cervical nodes. Chest wall lymphatics, especially from the breasts, drain to the axillae. Lung disease, therefore, rarely involves the axillary nodes.

SKIN

The early stages of sarcoidosis and primary tuberculosis are often accompanied by erythema nodosum: painful red indurated areas, usually on the shins; although occasionally more extensive, they fade through bruising. The most common cause of erythema nodosum is sarcoidosis.

EYES

Horner's syndrome (miosis (contraction of the pupil), enophthalmos (backward displacement of the eyeball in the orbit), lack of sweating on the affected side of the face and ptosis (drooping of the upper eyelid)) is usually due to involvement of the sympathetic chain on the posterior chest wall by a bronchial carcinoma.

EXAMINATION OF THE CHEST

Inspection of the chest wall

First look for any deformities of the chest wall. In 'barrel chest' the chest wall is held in hyperinflation. The normal 'bucket handle' action of the ribs moving upwards and outwards, pivoting at the spinous processes and the costal cartilages, is converted into a 'pump handle' up and down motion. Barrel chest is seen in states of chronic airflow limitation.

In pectus excavatum ('funnel chest'), the sternum is depressed. In pectus carinatum ('pigeon chest'), the sternum and costal cartilages project outwards.

Flattening of part of the chest can be due either to underlying lung disease (which usually has to be long-standing) or to scoliosis.

Kyphosis is forward curvature of the spine; scoliosis is a lateral curvature. Both, but scoliosis in particular, can lead to respiratory failure.

Air in the subcutaneous tissue is termed surgical emphysema. The tissues of the upper chest and neck are swollen, sometimes grossly so (Michelin man). The tissues have a characteristic crackling sensation on palpation. In pneumothorax, the air probably tracks from ruptured alveoli, through the root of the lungs to the mediastinum, thence up into the neck. On auscultation of the precordium, you may hear a curious extra sound in time with the heart (mediastinal crunch).

Breathing patterns

Note rate, depth and regularity. Does the chest move equally on the two sides?

You should note an increase in rate or depth. An increase in rate may occur in any severe lung disease. Patients with hyper-ventilation may breathe both faster and more deeply, although the increase can be subtle and easily missed. Patients with acidosis from renal failure, diabetic ketoacidosis and aspirin overdosage will have deep sighing (Kussmaul) respirations as they try to excrete carbon dioxide.

Cheyne–Stokes respiration is a waxing and waning of the respiratory depth over a minute or so from deep respirations to almost no breathing at all. It is often seen in patients with terminal disease.

The typical patient with airflow limitation has trouble breathing out. Inspiration may be brief, but expiration is a prolonged laboured manoeuvre. Many of these patients breathe out through pursed lips, as if they were whistling; this keeps open the distal airways to allow fuller, although longer, expiration.

Can the patient carry on a normal conversation or does he or she have to break up sentences, even perhaps to single words at a time? Patients with severe respiratory distress use their accessory muscles of respiration.

Wheeze is a prolonged expiratory noise, often audible to the patient as well as the doctor, and implies airflow limitation. Stridor is a harsh, chiefly inspiratory noise and implies obstruction in the central airways.

'PINK PUFFERS' AND 'BLUE BLOATERS'

The terms 'pink puffers' and 'blue bloaters' are applied to the overall appearances of some patients with chronic airflow limitation. 'Blue bloaters' are cyanosed from hypoxia and bloated from right-sided heart failure. 'Pink puffers' are not cyanosed and are thin. Investigation shows features associated with emphysema. Cough and sputum are less common, but the patients are breathless.

Palpation

Trachea and mediastinum

Start palpation by feeling for the position of the trachea by placing two fingers either side of the trachea and judging whether the distances between it and the sternomastoid tendons are equal on the two sides. The trachea gives an indication about the position of the mediastinum.

The position of the apex beat also gives information about the position of the mediastinum, as long as the heart is not enlarged.

Differential diagnosis
Mediastinal displacement

Away from the lesion
- Pneumothorax
- Effusion (large)

Towards the lesion
- Lung collapse from central airway obstruction
- Localised fibrosis

A systematic approach

Comparison is made between the two sides of the body as abnormality is likely to be confined to one side.

VOCAL FREMITUS

This is performed by placing either the edge or the flat of your hand on the chest and asking the patient to say 'ninety-nine' or count 'one, two, three'. The vibrations are transmitted through the lung substance and are felt by the hand. The test is the same as for vocal resonance.

CHEST EXPANSION

A good method is to put the fingers of both your hands as far round the chest as possible and then bring the thumbs together in the midline but to keep the thumbs off the chest wall. The patient is then asked to take a deep breath in; the chest wall, by moving outwards, moves the fingers outwards and the thumbs are in turn distracted away from the midline. The thumbs must be free: if they are also fixed to the chest wall they will not move.

Expansion can be reduced on both sides equally by severe airflow limitation, extensive generalised lung fibrosis and chest wall problems (e.g. ankylosing spondylitis).

Unilateral reduction implies that air cannot enter that side and is seen in pleural effusion, lung collapse, pneumothorax and pneumonia.

Percussion

Use both hands, placing the fingers of one hand on the chest with the fingers separated and strike one of them with the terminal phalynx of the middle finger of the other hand; it must be removed again immediately, like the clapper inside a bell. The striking movement should be a flick of the wrist and the striking finger should be at right angles to the other finger. As well as hearing the percussion note, vibrations will be felt by your hand on the chest wall. The finger on the chest should be parallel to the expected line of dullness. This will produce a clearly defined change in note from normal to dull. The apex of the lung can be examined by tapping directly on the middle of the clavicle.

Patients with overinflated lungs, particularly those with emphysema, have increased resonance. Resonance is decreased moderately in consolidation and fibrosis, and markedly if there is fluid between the lung and the chest wall, that is, stony dullness. A collapsed lobe can compress to a very small volume and compensatory overinflation of the other lobe fills the space. The percussion note may then be normal.

Percussion can also be used to determine movement of the diaphragm because the level of dullness will descend as the patient breathes in (tidal percussion). Dullness is expected over the liver, which anteriorly reaches as high as the sixth costal cartilage. Resonance here, again a subjective finding, implies increased air in the lungs and is common in overinflation and emphysema.

 Differential diagnosis
Dullness to percussion

Moderate
- Consolidation
- Fibrosis
- Collapse

'Stony'
- Pleural fluid

Auscultation

Ask the patient to take deep breaths through the mouth, then listen in sequence over the chest. Start at the apices and compare each side.

Breath sounds are termed either vesicular or bronchial and the added sounds are divided into crackles, wheezes and rubs.

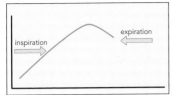

Fig. 5.5 Timing of vesicular breathing.

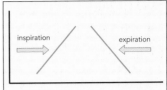

Fig. 5.6 Timing of bronchial breathing.

VESICULAR BREATH SOUNDS

This is the sound heard over normal lungs and is heard on inspiration and the first part of expiration (Fig. 5.5). Reduction in vesicular breath sounds can be expected with airways obstruction as in asthma, emphysema or tumour. The breath sounds can be strikingly reduced in emphysema.

BRONCHIAL BREATHING

Traditionally, bronchial breathing is described by its timing as occurring in both inspiration and expiration with a gap in between (Fig. 5.6). Concentrate on the essential feature, the quality of the sound. It can be mimicked to some extent by listening over the trachea with the stethoscope.

The main cause of bronchial breathing is consolidation. Lung abscess, if near the chest wall, can cause bronchial breathing, because of the consolidation around it. Dense fibrosis is an occasional cause. Breath sounds over an effusion will be diminished but bronchial breathing may be heard over its upper level, because the effusion compresses the lung.

VOCAL RESONANCE

This is the auscultatory equivalent of vocal fremitus. Place the stethoscope on the chest and ask the patient to say 'ninety-nine'. Normally the sound produced is 'fuzzy'. The sound is increased in consolidation (better transmission through solid lung) and decreased if there is air, fluid or pleural thickening between the lung and the chest wall. The changes of vocal fremitus are the same. Sometimes the increased transmission of sound is so marked that even when the patient whispers, the sound is still heard clearly over the affected lung (whispering pectoriloquy).

ADDED SOUNDS
Wheezes

These are prolonged musical sounds largely occurring on expiration, sometimes on inspiration. A single wheeze can occur and may then suggest a single narrowing, often caused by a carcinoma or foreign body (fixed wheeze).

Wheezes are typical of airway narrowing from any cause. Asthma and chronic bronchitis are the most common.

Wheeze-like breath sounds can disappear in severe asthma and emphysema because of low rates of airflow.

 Emergency
Signs of asthma in adults

Signs of acute severe asthma in adults
- Unable to complete sentences
- Pulse >110 beats/min
- Respirations >25 breaths/min
- Peak flow <50% predicted or best

Signs of life-threatening asthma in adults
- Silent chest
- Cyanosis
- Bradycardia
- Exhaustion
- Peak flow <33% predicted or best

Stridor

Stridor may be heard better without a stethoscope by putting your ear close to the patient's mouth, asking the patient to breathe in and out. It is a sign of large airway narrowing in the larynx, trachea or main bronchi.

Crackles

The sound of 'fine' crackles can be imitated by rolling the hairs of your temple together between your fingers. They occur in inspiration and are high-pitched, explosive sound. Conditions that largely involve the alveoli, such as left ventricular failure, fibrosis and pneumonia, tend to produce crackles later on inspiration.

 Differential diagnosis
Crackles

- Left ventricular failure
- Fibrosing alveolitis
- Extrinsic allergic alveolitis
- Pneumonia
- Bronchiectasis
- Chronic bronchitis
- Asbestosis

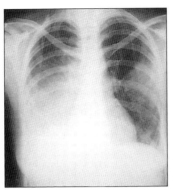

Mediastinum central
Expansion ↓
Percussion note ↓
Breath sounds bronchial
Whispering pectoriloquy
Crackles
Pleural rub

Fig. 5.7 Consolidation (unusual because it affects both lungs).

Note whether the crackles are localised. This would be expected in pneumonia and mild cases of bronchiectasis. Pulmonary oedema and fibrosing alveolitis typically affect both lung bases equally.

Normal people, especially smokers, may have a few basal crackles; these often clear with a few deep breaths.

Pleural rub

This is caused by the inflamed surfaces of the pleura rubbing together. Rubs are usually heard on both inspiration and expiration. If there is any pain, ask the patient to point to the site of the pain; this often localises the rub too. Rubs are heard in all varieties of pleural inflammation, such as in pneumonia and pulmonary embolism.

COMMON PATTERNS OF ABNORMALITY

Consolidation

Inspection of the chest may show diminished movement on the affected side; palpation shows no shift of the mediastinum but expansion is reduced, vocal fremitus may be increased, percussion note will be moderately impaired, breath sounds will be bronchial over the affected area with whispering pectoriloquy and there may be a pleural rub. Early and late in the disease process there may also be crackles. In lobar pneumonia, the changes are localised to a lobe. More widespread changes suggest 'bronchopneumonia' or 'atypical pneumonia' caused by viruses, mycoplasma and other organisms (Fig. 5.7).

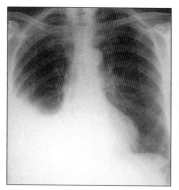

Mediastinum usually central
Expansion ↓
Percussion ↓
Breath sounds ↓
Sometimes bronchial
    breathing or a pleural
    rub at upper level

Fig. 5.8 Small effusion.

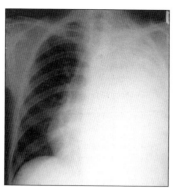

Mediastinum displaced
Expansion ↓
Percussion ↓
Breath sounds ↓

Fig. 5.9 Large effusion.

Pleural fluid

Expansion is diminished on the affected side, vocal fremitus is reduced, percussion note is markedly reduced, ('stony dullness'), and breath sounds are absent or markedly reduced (Fig. 5.8). Bronchial breathing may be heard at the upper level of the effusion (Fig. 5.9).

Pneumothorax

The affected side moves less well, vocal fremitus is reduced and the percussion note is normal. The expected increased resonance can be difficult to detect and it is the conjunction of diminished breath sounds with a normal percussion note that distinguishes it from other causes

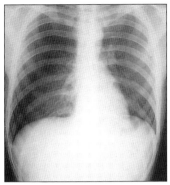

Mediastinum sometimes
   displaced
Expansion ↓
Percussion normal or ↑
Breath sounds ↓
No added sounds

Fig. 5.10   Pneumothorax on right.

Risk factors
Some causes of pneumothorax

- No cause found
- Apical blebs
- Chronic bronchitis and emphysema
- Staphylococcal pneumonia

- Asthma
- Tuberculosis
- Cystic fibrosis
- Trauma

of diminished breath sounds when there is also dullness to percussion. Vocal resonance is reduced and there are no added sounds (Fig. 5.10).

Chronic airflow limitation

There may be hyperinflation of the chest, pursed lip breathing and use of accessory muscles of respiration. Expansion may well be reduced but usually equally so. Vocal fremitus is normal, percussion is usually normal but there may be increased resonance and reduced hepatic and cardiac dullness. Breath sounds are vesicular and sometimes reduced; the added sounds are wheezes and often crackles (Fig. 5.11).

Lung and lobar collapse

There is diminished movement on the affected side, with the mediastinum deviating to that side. The percussion note is markedly reduced if the whole lung is involved. Breath sounds are diminished

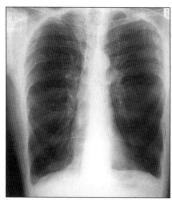

Hyperinflation
Mediastinum central
Hepatic and cardiac
    dullness ↓
Vesicular breath sounds
Wheezes and crackles
Radiograph often normal
    but here shows
    overinflation and low
    flat diaphragms

Fig. 5.11 Chronic airflow limitation.

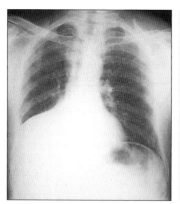

Mediastinum displaced
Expansion reduced
Percussion normal or ↓
Breath sounds vesicular
    but ↓ or sometimes
    bronchial

Fig. 5.12 Right, middle and lower lobe collapse.

but remain vesicular in lobar collapse and may be absent if the whole lung is involved. Vocal resonance is decreased. As already indicated, bronchial breathing, increased vocal resonance and whispering pectoriloquy can be heard in upper lobe collapse because of direct transmission of sound from the trachea. Bronchial breathing is also heard in collapse of other lobes if the airways remain patent (Fig. 5.12).

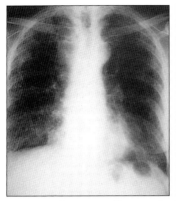

Mediastinum central
Expansion equally ↓
Percussion normal or ↓
Breath sounds vesicular
(occasionally bronchial)
Crackles

Fig. 5.13 Cryptogenic fibrosing alveolitis.

Lung fibrosis

Localised changes produce similar signs to lung collapse. Generalised disease is best illustrated by cryptogenic fibrosing alveolitis. The lungs are stiff, expansion may be reduced, but equally, and the mediastinum is central. Vocal fremitus is normal, percussion note is normal or slightly reduced, breath sounds are vesicular, although occasionally bronchial, yet there are marked crackles, initially confined to the bases but later extending up the chest (Fig. 5.13).

 Examination of elderly people
Respiratory examination

- Be aware of multiple problems
- Occupational history still valid
  - mesothelioma occurs long after exposure
  - pneumoconiosis changes persist for life
- Not all breathless elderly patients have chronic obstructive pulmonary disease
- Respiratory and cardiac disease often coexist
- Right ventricular failure as a consequence of lung disease is difficult to distinguish from congestive cardiac failure
- Disability may be multifactorial

Review
Framework for the routine examination of the respiratory system

1. While taking the history, watch for respiratory distress, particularly while talking. Note any clues from the patient's surroundings
2. Look at the hands for clubbing, cyanosis and evidence of carbon dioxide retention
3. Look at the mucous membranes for central cyanosis
4. Check the jugular venous pulse for evidence of cor pulmonale
5. Palpate for supraclavicular lymph nodes
6. Inspect the chest wall for deformities and inequalities
7. Note the pattern of breathing
8. Palpate the trachea for any displacement
9. Palpate the front of the chest for vocal fremitus and for right ventricular hypertrophy
10. Assess expansion of the chest from the front and note any inequalities
11. Percuss the front of the chest, comparing one side with the other and noting any areas of dullness; include the axillae
12. Auscultate the chest similarly and decide on the presence and nature of the breath sounds
13. Test for vocal resonance and, where appropriate, whispering pectoriloquy
14. Note any added sounds
15. Repeat last six steps on the back of the chest
16. If appropriate, measure the peak flow rate

6.
The Heart and Cardiovascular System

CLINICAL HISTORY

Breathlessness

Patients with heart disease that causes breathlessness experience it during physical exertion (exertional dyspnoea) and sometimes when they lie flat in bed (positional dyspnoea or orthopnoea). Sometimes, the patient awakes from sleep extremely breathless and has to sit up gasping for breath (paroxysmal nocturnal dyspnoea).

Differential diagnosis
Dyspnoea

- Heart failure
- Ischaemic heart disease (atypical angina)
- Lung disease
- Severe anaemia

Questions to ask
Breathlessness

- Do you ever feel short of breath?
- Does this happen on exertion?
- How much can you do before getting breathless?
- Do you ever wake up gasping for breath?
- If so, do you have to sit up or get out of bed?
- How many pillows do you sleep on?
- Do you cough or wheeze when you are short of breath?

Symptoms and signs
New York Heart Association classification of heart failure

Grade

I   No symptoms at rest, dyspnoea only on vigorous exertion

II   No symptoms at rest, dyspnoea on moderate exertion

III   May be mild symptoms at rest, dyspnoea on mild exertion, severe dyspnoea on moderate exertion

IV   Significant dyspnoea at rest, severe dyspnoea even on very mild exertion. Patient often bed bound

Chest pain

CHEST PAIN CAUSED BY MYOCARDIAL ISCHAEMIA

The most common type of chest pain associated with heart disease is called angina pectoris. Most patients with angina have a narrowing or stenosis in one or more coronary arteries. Less often, angina is a symptom of aortic stenosis or hypertrophic cardiomyopathy.

Questions to ask
Angina

- Do you get pain in your chest on exertion (e.g. climbing stairs)?
- Whereabouts in the chest do you feel it?
- Is it worse in cold weather?
- Is it worse if you exercise after a big meal?
- Is it bad enough to stop you from exercising?
- Does it go away when you rest?
- Do you ever get similar pain if you get excited or upset?

Symptoms and signs
Anginal pain

- Brought on by physical or emotional exertion
- Relieved by rest
- Usually crushing, squeezing or constricting in nature
- Usually retrosternal
- Often worse after food or in cold winds
- Often relieved by nitrates

Differential diagnosis
Chest pain at rest

- Myocardial infarction
- Unstable angina
- Dissecting aortic aneurysm
- Oesophageal pain
- Pericarditis
- Pleuritic pain
- Musculoskeletal pain
- Herpes zoster (shingles)

PERICARDITIS

The patient characteristically complains of pain that is usually described as a constant soreness behind the breast bone and that often gets much worse if the patient takes a deep breath. Unlike the pain of angina or myocardial infarction, pericarditic pain is related to movement but not to physical exertion. It sometimes radiates to the tip of the left shoulder.

MUSCULOSKELETAL CHEST PAIN

Characteristically, it tends to be an aching pain, the onset of which may relate to a particular twist or movement. There is often localised tenderness, particularly over the costal cartilages.

DISSECTING AORTIC ANEURYSM

Dissecting aneurysm of the thoracic aorta causes a rare form of chest pain that usually starts as a 'tearing' sensation, often felt most between the shoulder blades or in the back. The pain is usually severe and persistent and may be mistaken for the pain of myocardial infarction.

OTHER CHEST PAINS

Other chest pains that may masquerade as cardiac pain include the pain of pleurisy, of an acute pneumothorax or of shingles.

PALPITATION

Palpitation is defined as abnormal awareness of the heart beat. It is often helpful to ask the patient to tap out the heart rhythm on the table.

Questions to ask
Palpitation

- Please could you tap out on the table the rate you think your heart goes at during an attack?
- Is the heart beat regular or irregular?
- Is there anything that sets attacks off?
- Can you do anything to stop an attack?
- What do you do when you have an attack?
- Are there any foods that seem to make symptoms worse?
- What medicines are you taking?

Differential diagnosis
Palpitation

- Extrasystoles
- Paroxysmal atrial fibrillation
- Paroxysmal supraventricular tachycardia
- Thyrotoxicosis
- Perimenopausal

SYNCOPE (FAINTING, BLACKOUTS)

Syncope is defined as loss of consciousness resulting from a transient failure of blood supply to the brain. The main differential diagnosis is from epilepsy. The common causes of syncope are simple fainting (vasovagal syncope), its variants such as micturition syncope, postural hypotension, vertebrobasilar insufficiency and cardiac arrhythmias, particularly intermittent heart block.

In fainting, loss of consciousness is seldom abrupt; the patient looks pale both before and immediately afterwards. In contrast, syncope caused by heart block is often sudden, unheralded and complete. The patient looks pale while collapsed, recovery (which is often equally sudden) may be heralded by a pink flush. Vertebrobasilar insufficiency is common in elderly patients: there may be restricted neck movement and active or passive movements of the neck may precipitate symptoms.

CLAUDICATION

Intermittent claudication is the name given to a condition in which the patient experiences pain in one or both legs on walking and which eases up when the patient rests. The pain is usually an aching pain felt in the calf, thigh or buttocks.

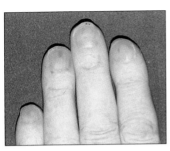

Fig. 6.1 Splinter haemorrhage in the ring finger of a man with infective endocarditis. There is an older, fading 'splinter' under the nail of the index finger. Splinter haemorrhages are often smaller and darker than this.

A FRAMEWORK FOR THE ROUTINE PHYSICAL EXAMINATION OF THE CARDIOVASCULAR SYSTEM

Hands in heart disease

The fingernails may show splinter haemorrhages (Fig. 6.1) in subacute infective endocarditis and finger clubbing in endocarditis or cyanotic congenital heart disease.

Feeling the peripheral pulses

The right radial pulse is used to assess heart rate and rhythm. It is not a good pulse from which to attempt to assess pulse character. In patients with suspected coarctation of the aorta, it is helpful simultaneously to feel the radial and the femoral pulse. In coarctation not only is the volume of the femoral pulse diminished but it is also appreciably delayed compared with the radial pulse.

BRACHIAL PULSE

Use the thumb of the right hand, applied to the front of the elbow just medial to the biceps tendon with the fingers cupped round the back of the elbow. Figure 6.2 illustrates the different pulse waveforms.

CAROTID PULSE

The best way to feel the patient's right carotid artery is to locate the tip of the examiner's left thumb against the patient's larynx (Fig. 6.3). In severe aortic stenosis, there is characteristically a slow rising carotid pulse. Another sign best appreciated at the carotid is the jerky pulse of hypertrophic cardiomyopathy.

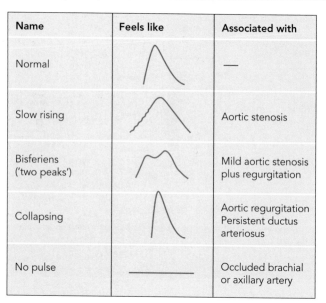

Name	Feels like	Associated with
Normal		—
Slow rising		Aortic stenosis
Bisferiens ('two peaks')		Mild aortic stenosis plus regurgitation
Collapsing		Aortic regurgitation Persistent ductus arteriosus
No pulse		Occluded brachial or axillary artery

Fig. 6.2 Different pulse waveforms are associated with different cardiac or vascular abnormalities.

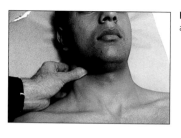

Fig. 6.3 Palpation of the carotid artery using the thumb.

FEMORAL PULSE

This is best examined by placing the thumb or finger directly above the superior public ramus and midway between the pubic tubercle and anterior superior iliac spine.

POPLITEAL PULSE

The popliteal pulse is readily felt by compressing it against the posterior surface of the distal end of the femur. The patient lies flat with the knee slightly flexed. The fingers of one hand are used to press the tips of the fingers of the other hand into the popliteal fossa to feel the popliteal artery against the back of the knee joint.

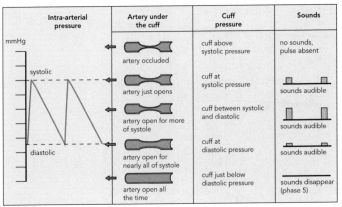

	Intra-arterial pressure	Artery under the cuff	Cuff pressure	Sounds
mmHg		artery occluded	cuff above systolic pressure	no sounds, pulse absent
systolic		artery just opens	cuff at systolic pressure	sounds audible
		artery open for more of systole	cuff between systolic and diastolic	sounds audible
diastolic		artery open for nearly all of systole	cuff at diastolic pressure	sounds audible
		artery open all the time	cuff just below diastolic pressure	sounds disappear (phase 5)

Fig. 6.4 The relationship between cuff pressure, Korotkoff sounds and arterial pressure.

DORSALIS PEDIS AND TIBIALIS POSTERIOR PULSES

The dorsalis pedis pulse is felt with the fingers aligned along the dorsum of the foot lateral to the extensor hallucis longus tendon; the tibialis posterior pulse is felt with the fingers cupped round the ankle just posterior to the medial malleolus.

Measuring blood pressure

The generation of the Korotkoff sounds is shown diagrammatically in Figure 6.4.

Check the systolic pressure roughly by palpation of the radial artery before applying the stethoscope. Pressure in the cuff should be reduced slowly, at about 1 mmHg/s.

Patients with very high blood pressure often have other evidence of hypertensive disease in the form of retinal changes, left ventricular hypertrophy and proteinuria. Most authorities would accept a phase 5 diastolic pressure of over 100 mmHg on repeated measurement as defining a hypertensive population. A diastolic pressure of greater than 120 mmHg and evidence of end organ damage would define patients with severe hypertension.

The converse of hypertension is hypotension. Although a systolic blood pressure of less than 100 mmHg is part of the definition of shock, hypotension is usually defined by its consequences (e.g. impaired cerebral or renal function) rather than by some arbitary pressure level. Some patients have postural hypotension, which most commonly manifests as dizziness when the patient attempts to stand upright. The diagnosis is made by measuring the blood pressure with the patient lying and standing.

Differential diagnosis
Systemic hypertension

- Primary 'essential' hypertension
- Secondary: Aortic coarctation
- Hormonal: Congenital
                 – adrenal hyperplasia
                 – 11-hydroxylase deficiency
                 Acquired
                 – phaeochromocytoma
                 – Conn's syndrome
                 – Cushing's syndrome
- Renal: Polycystic kidneys
                 Renal artery stenosis
                 Acute glomerulonephritis
                 Chronic renal disease
- Drug-related: Steroids
                 Contraceptive pill
                 Nonsteroidal anti-inflammatory drugs
                 Ciclosporin

Differential diagnosis
Hypotension

Impaired cardiac output
- Myocardial infarction
- Pericardial tamponade
- Massive pulmonary embolism
- Acute valve incompetence

Hypovolaemia
- Haemorrhage
- Diabetic precoma
- Dehydration from diarrhoea or vomiting

Excessive vasodilatation
- Anaphylaxis
- Gram-negative septicaemia
- Drugs
- Autonomic failure

Emergency
Severe hypotension (shock)

Emergency medical assessment of the patient with severe hypotension (shock)

1. **History** (from patient, relatives or attendants)
   - Has there been any trauma, haemorrhage or substance abuse?
   - Has onset been sudden or gradual (over hours or days, e.g. diabetic ketoacidosis, dysentery)?
   - Has there been any pain (i) in the chest (myocardial infarction, dissecting aneurysm) or (ii) elsewhere (e.g. headache in meningococcal septicaemia)?
   - Is there any other relevant history (e.g. bed rest, airline travel in massive pulmonary embolism)?

2. **Clinical examination**
   - Before starting the examination, check that the patient's airway is safe and, if possible, attach an ECG monitor
   - Check whether the patient is more comfortable sitting up (think of pulmonary oedema) or lying flat (think of hypovolaemia or pulmonary embolism)
   - Remove external clothes and conduct a quick but thorough examination for signs of trauma or haemorrhage if appropriate. Usually the skin in shock is pale and cold but if it is warm or red think of septicaemia or allergy
   - Assess the pulse. Normally it would be fast (100–120 beats/min) in shock; if very slow think of heart block; if more rapid consider an arrhythmia
   - Quickly assess the major pulses (carotid, femorals). If asymmetrical, think of dissecting aortic aneurysm
   - Try and assess the jugular venous pressure. A very high jugular venous pressure suggests pulmonary embolism or cardiac tamponade
   - Check that the trachea is central and that air entry can be heard on both sides of the chest (if not, think of tension pneumothorax). If there are widespread crackles in the lungs, think of pulmonary oedema
   - Listen to the front of the chest for murmurs or abnormal heart sounds (often very difficult if the heart rate is rapid)
   - Gently palpate the abdomen for tenderness or pulsation (think of ruptured aortic aneurysm)
   - If appropriate consider rectal or vaginal examination for hidden haemorrhage

Emergency
Severe hypotension (shock) – *(cont'd)*

3. Investigation

- As soon as possible record an ECG (diagnosis of myocardial infarction, arrhythmia, pulmonary embolism) and take a chest radiograph (and if appropriate other radiographs, for example, in the case of trauma). Consider emergency echocardiography if diagnosis is still in doubt

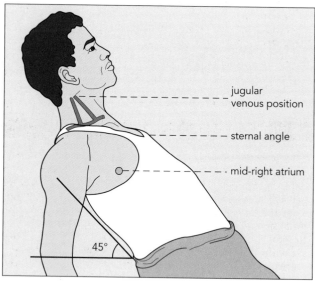

Fig. 6.5 Relationship of the jugular venous pulsation, right atrium and manubriosternal angle.

EVALUATION OF THE JUGULAR VENOUS PULSE

When the patient is standing or sitting upright, the internal jugular vein is collapsed, and when the patient is lying flat, it is completely filled. If the patient lies supine at approximately 45°, the point at which jugular venous pulsation becomes visible is usually just above the clavicle; this is the position usually chosen for examination of the jugular venous pulse. It is usual to express the height of jugular venous pulsation above the manubriosternal angle (Fig. 6.5). A normal jugular venous pressure is less than 4 cm above the manubriosternal angle.

By far the most common cause of a raised jugular venous pressure is congestive heart failure, in which the raised venous pressure reflects the right ventricular failure component. A raised but nonpulsatile jugular venous pressure should bring to mind the possibility of superior vena cava obstruction.

Differential diagnosis
Raised jugular venous pressure

- Congestive or right-sided heart failure
- Tricuspid reflux
- Pericardial tamponade
- Pulmonary embolism
- Iatrogenic fluid overload
- Superior vena cava obstruction

PALPATION OF THE PRECORDIUM

Palpate the precordium by laying the flat of the hand and the outstretched fingers on the chest wall to the left of the sternum. First locate the 'apex beat'. This is the furthest outward and downward point at which pulsation is easily palpable. The normal adult apex beat with the patient lying supine at 45° is the fifth or sixth left intercostal space, in the midclavicular line.

A forceful apex beat usually indicates increased cardiac output. A diffuse poorly localised apex beat is commonly found after damage to the ventricular muscle, either by myocardial infarction or as a result of cardiomyopathy. This diffuse impulse can often be seen as well as felt by inspecting the precordium. The character of the cardiac impulse in left ventricular hypertrophy is distinctive, being a sustained and forceful heave rather than a short sharp impulse. In mitral stenosis, the cardiac apex is often described as tapping. Right

Differential diagnosis
Left ventricular hypertrophy

- Hypertension
- Aortic stenosis
- Hypertrophic cardiomyopathy

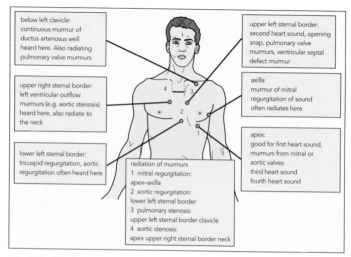

below left clavicle:
continuous murmur of
ductus arteriosus well
heard here. Also radiating
pulmonary valve murmurs

upper left sternal border:
second heart sound, opening
snap, pulmonary valve
murmurs, ventricular septal
defect murmur

upper right sternal border:
left ventricular outflow
murmurs (e.g. aortic stenosis)
heard here, also radiate to
the neck

axilla:
murmur of mitral
regurgitation of sound
often radiates here

lower left sternal border:
tricuspid regurgitation, aortic
regurgitation often heard here

apex:
good for first heart sound,
murmurs from mitral or
aortic valves
third heart sound
fourth heart sound

radiation of murmurs
1 mitral regurgitation:
apex–axilla
2 aortic regurgitation:
lower left sternal border
3 pulmonary stenosis:
upper left sternal border clavicle
4 aortic stenosis:
apex upper right sternal border neck

Fig. 6.6 Cardiac auscultation; the best sites for hearing sounds and murmurs depend on where the sound is produced and to where turbulent blood flows radiate.

ventricular hypertrophy or dilatation is felt as a heave close to the left sternal border.

While palpating the heart, the examining hand will sometimes detect a vibration or 'thrill'. Systolic thrills may accompany aortic stenosis, ventricular septal defect or mitral reflex.

AUSCULTATION OF THE HEART

The bell is central for listening to low-pitched sounds such as the mid-diastolic murmur of mitral stenosis or the third heart sound of cardiac failure. The diaphragm filters out low-pitched sounds and emphasises high-pitched ones. The diaphragm is best for analysing the second heart sound, ejection and mid-systolic clicks and the soft but high-pitched early diastolic murmur of aortic regurgitation.

When auscultating the heart, you should listen at the apex, at the base (the part of the heart between the apex and the sternum) and in the aortic and pulmonary areas to the right and left of the sternum, respectively (Fig. 6.6).

Heart sounds

FIRST AND SECOND HEART SOUNDS

 Differential diagnosis
Factors that may influence the intensity of the heart sounds

Loud first sound
- Hyperdynamic circulation (fever, exercise)
- Mitral stenosis
- Atrial myxoma (rare)

Soft first sound
- Low cardiac output (rest, heart failure)
- Tachycardia
- Severe mitral reflux (caused by destruction of valve)

Variable intensity of first sound
- Atrial fibrillation
- Complete heart block

Loud aortic component of second sound
- Systemic hypertension
- Dilated aortic root

Soft aortic component of second sound
- Calcific aortic stenosis

Loud pulmonary component of second sound
- Pulmonary hypertension

THIRD AND FOURTH HEART SOUNDS

The third heart sound is a low-pitched, thudding sound that occurs in diastole and coincides with the end of the rapid phase of ventricular filling. A physiological third heart sound occurs in young fit adults under circumstances of increased cardiac output (e.g. in athletes, in the presence of a fever or during pregnancy). A pathological third heart sound is usually a marker for severe impairment of left ventricular function. It can be heard in dilated cardiomyopathy, after acute myocardial infarction or in acute massive pulmonary embolism. In patients with a pathological third heart sound, there is nearly always a tachycardia and the first and second heart sounds are relatively quiet. The cadence of first, second and third heart sounds therefore sounds something like 'da-da-boom, da-da-boom' and has been given the name of a gallop rhythm.

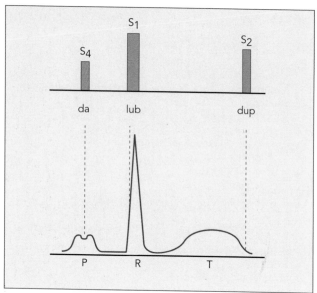

Fig. 6.7 The fourth heart sound.

A fourth heart sound is an extra heart sound that coincides with atrial contraction. It is usually best heard in patients whose left atrium is hypertrophied (e.g. as a consequence of systemic hypertension or hypertrophic cardiomyopathy). A fourth sound sounds a little like 'da-lup-dup, da-lub-dup' (Fig. 6.7).

OTHER EXTRA HEART SOUNDS

Ejection click A high-pitched ringing sound usually follows very shortly after the first heart sound (Fig. 6.8). It is a feature of aortic or pulmonary valve stenosis, caused by the sudden opening of the deformed valve.

Opening snap A diastolic sound heard in mitral stenosis and associated with the tensing of the diaphragm formed by the stenosed mitral valve, it is best heard to the left of the sternum and sounds rather like the second part of a widely split second heart sound.

Mid-systolic clicks These are usually associated with mitral valve prolapse and are caused by the tensing of the long and redundant chordae tendineae of these valves. The clicks may or may not be associated with a late systolic murmur.

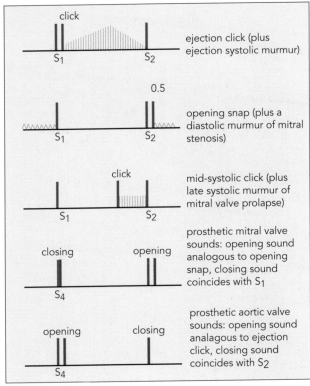

Fig. 6.8 Extra heart sounds.

Sounds from artificial heart valves The ball, disc or poppet in an artificial heart valve usually makes a noise both when it opens and when the valve closes.

MURMURS

The important point in analysing a murmur is where it occurs in the cardiac cycle.

Systolic murmurs Murmurs that are due to leakage of blood through an incompetent mitral or tricuspid valve or a ventricular septal defect are usually of similar intensity throughout the length of systole. They are called pansystolic or holosystolic murmurs (Fig. 6.9). Occasionally, a valve is competent at the start of systole but starts to leak half way through. This is common in patients with mitral valve

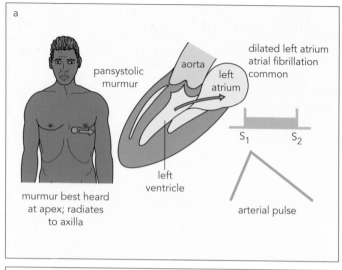

a

pansystolic
murmur

aorta

left
atrium

dilated left atrium
atrial fibrillation
common

left
ventricle

S_1 S_2

murmur best heard
at apex; radiates
to axilla

arterial pulse

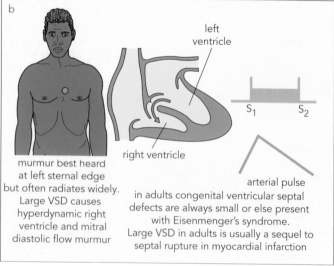

b

left
ventricle

right ventricle

S_1 S_2

murmur best heard
at left sternal edge
but often radiates widely.
Large VSD causes
hyperdynamic right
ventricle and mitral
diastolic flow murmur

arterial pulse

in adults congenital ventricular septal
defects are always small or else present
with Eisenmenger's syndrome.
Large VSD in adults is usually a sequel to
septal rupture in myocardial infarction

Fig. 6.9 Pansystolic (holosystolic) murmurs: (a) mitral regurgitation;
(b) ventricular septal defect.

Symptoms and signs
Grading the intensity of murmurs

- Grade 1 – just audible with a good stethoscope in a quiet room
- Grade 2 – quiet but readily audible with a stethoscope
- Grade 3 – easily heard with a stethoscope
- Grade 4 – a loud, obvious murmur
- Grade 5 – very loud, heard not only over the precordium but elsewhere in the body

prolapse. The result is a murmur that starts in mid- or late systole and is called a mid-systolic or late systolic murmur, respectively.

Murmurs due to blood being forced through a narrow aortic or pulmonary valve or to increased blood flow through a normal aortic or pulmonary valve tend to start quietly at the beginning of systole, rise to a crescendo in mid-systole and then become quiet again towards the end of systole. Such murmurs are called ejection systolic murmurs (Fig. 6.10).

Innocent murmurs   Innocent murmurs are murmurs that are not associated with any major structural abnormality in the heart. They are common in children and young adults. They have the following characteristics: always systolic and always quiet (less than grade 3); usually best heard at the left sternal edge; no associated ventricular hypertrophy; and normal heart sounds, pulses, chest radiograph and ECG.

Diastolic murmurs   An early diastolic murmur (Fig. 6.11) is nearly always caused by incompetence of either the aortic or the pulmonary valve. It is maximal at the beginning of diastole when aortic or pulmonary pressure is highest and rapidly becomes quieter (decrescendo) as pressure in the great vessel falls.

A mid-diastolic murmur is usually caused by either blood flow through a narrowed mitral or tricuspid valve or, occasionally, to increased blood flow through one of these valves (e.g. in children with atrial septal defect). The characteristic murmur of mitral stenosis is a low-pitched, rumbling murmur heard throughout diastole (Fig. 6.12). In patients in sinus rhythm, it gets louder just before the onset of systole as a result of atrial contraction increasing blood flow through the narrowed valve. Sometimes patients with aortic reflux have a mid-diastolic murmur. This is caused by the regurgitant blood from the incompetent aortic valve setting up a vibration of the anterior leaflet of the mitral valve (Austin Flint murmur).

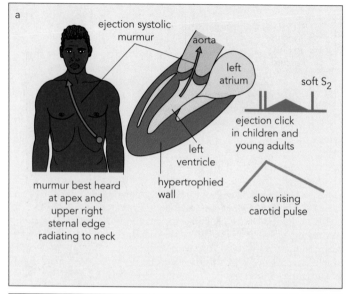

a

ejection systolic murmur

aorta

left atrium

soft S₂

left ventricle

ejection click in children and young adults

murmur best heard at apex and upper right sternal edge radiating to neck

hypertrophied wall

slow rising carotid pulse

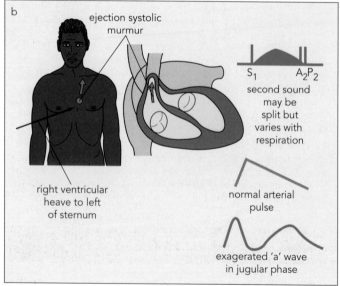

b

ejection systolic murmur

S_1 $A_2 P_2$

second sound may be split but varies with respiration

right ventricular heave to left of sternum

normal arterial pulse

exaggerated 'a' wave in jugular phase

Fig. 6.10 Ejection systolic murmurs: (a) aortic stenosis; (b) pulmonary stenosis.

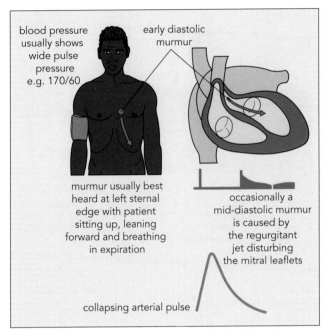

Fig. 6.11 Aortic regurgitation as an example of an early diastolic murmur.

The murmur of mitral stenosis is best heard if the patient is rolled onto his or her left side and the stethoscope bell applied to the cardiac apex. The murmur of aortic reflux is sometimes best heard if the patient is made to sit up, lean forward and breathe out fully while the stethoscope is applied at the left side of the lower part of the sternum.

Systolic murmurs arising at the pulmonary valve (i.e. pulmonary stenosis flow murmurs) tend to get louder during inspiration and quieter during expiration. Conversely, murmurs arising on the left side of the heart tend to get quieter during inspiration.

CARDIOVASCULAR SYSTEM AND CHEST EXAMINATION

The most important feature to look for in a patient with cardiac disease is the presence of crackles at the lung bases. These occur during inspiration and are an early sign of pulmonary oedema.

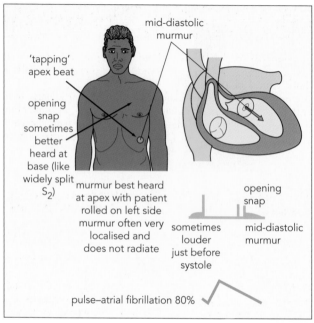

Fig. 6.12 Mitral stenosis as an example of a mid-diastolic murmur.

Dx Differential diagnosis
Sites of radiation of murmurs

Cause	'Primary site'	Radiation
Tricuspid regurgitation	Lower left sternal edge	Lower right sternal edge, liver
Pulmonary stenosis	Upper left sternal edge	Towards left clavicle, beneath left scapula
Mitral regurgitation	Apex	Left axilla, beneath left scapula
Aortic regurgitation	Left sternal edge	Down left sternal edge towards apex
Aortic stenosis	Apex	Towards upper right edge sternal edge, over carotids
Ventricular septal defect	Left sternal edge	All over pericardium
Mitral stenosis	Apex	Does not radiate

CARDIOVASCULAR SYSTEM AND ABDOMINAL EXAMINATION

In patients with tricuspid reflex, there is a marked hepatic pulsation in time with the regurgitation waves in the jugular venous pulse and with the arterial pulse.

Aneurysm of the abdominal aorta is common, particularly in men over the age of 60 years. The characteristic finding on examination is pulsation at about the level of the umbilicus. The characteristic features of an aneurysm are that it is enlarged in comparison with a normal aorta and that the pulsation it generates is expansile.

PERIPHERAL VASCULAR SYSTEM

Oedema

The oedema of heart failure is largely the result of increased venous pressure.

Peripheral oedema is usually a feature of right-sided heart failure or congestive heart failure. It characteristically accumulates at the lowest part of the body ('dependent oedema') in ambulant patients and the sacrum in patients confined to bed.

Oedema is detected in peripheral tissue by swelling that can be displaced by firm finger pressure and which leaves a pit when the finger is removed.

CLINICAL FEATURES OR SPECIFIC CARDIAC CONDITIONS

Heart failure

ACUTE HEART FAILURE

The most common manifestation of acute heart failure is a low systemic blood pressure. Acute left heart failure is accompanied by pulmonary oedema. The patient becomes extremely breathless, develops a cough and may produce frothy pink-stained sputum. The characteristic clinical sign of pulmonary oedema is widespread crepitations or crackling sounds, usually best heard at the base of the lungs.

CHRONIC HEART FAILURE

 Symptoms and signs
Chronic heart failure

- Fatigue on minimal exertion
- Exertional dyspnoea
- Peripheral oedema
- Abdominal discomfort (from hepatic distension)
- Nocturia (reversal of diurnal rhythm)
- Weight loss and cachexia

Coronary artery disease

ANGINA

Coronary artery disease has three principal manifestations: angina, acute myocardial infarction and chronic heart failure. Physical examination of the angina patient is frequently entirely normal. Nonetheless, the examiner should be alert for features of hyperlipidaemia, such as corneal arcus, thickened Achilles tendons and xanthelasma.

 Risk factors
Coronary artery disease

Inherited
- Familial hyperlipidaemia
- High lipoprotein a
- Others[1]

Acquired
- Smoking
- Acquired hyperlipidaemia
- Diabetes
- Hypertension
- Physical inactivity

[1]This includes many **common** polymorphisms with small (but cumulative) effects and some **rare** polymorphisms (e.g. pseudoxanthoma elasticum) with large effects.

MYOCARDIAL INFARCTION

The most characteristic symptom of myocardial infarction is chest pain, which is similar in distribution to the pain of angina but is usually much more severe and persists even when the patient rests. In a small proportion of patients, particularly elderly people and individuals with diabetes mellitus, myocardial infarction can be relatively painless.

PERIPHERAL VASCULAR DISEASE

Acute arterial obstruction presents with a cold, white, painful, pulseless limb. It is important to check pulses in the other limbs as well, even if they are not obviously ischaemic. Embolism to multiple sites may be the first clue to a cardiac disease such as atrial myxoma.

Chronic arterial insufficiency usually presents as intermittent claudication. The patient is aware of pain, in the leg, the thigh or the buttock, which comes on with walking and goes away when stopping to rest. Examination of the leg reveals weak or absent foot, knee and sometimes femoral pulses. There may be a murmur or bruit over the femoral artery. As the disease progresses, pain comes on with progressively less exertion until finally the patient experiences pain at rest. Pain is often worse at night. The skin tends to become discoloured and shiny, and hair is lost from the foot. Infection, which often starts with a small injury such as one derived from paring the toenails, spreads rapidly. Eventually, gangrene may affect the toes and foot.

Diseases of the peripheral veins

VARICOSE VEINS

Varicose veins are excessively dilated superficial leg veins. They are always most apparent when the patient is standing upright, and empty completely when the legs are raised above heart level. By elevating the legs to empty the veins and then watching the veins fill as the leg is lowered, it is often possible to see the sites of incompetent perforating veins and to control them by local finger pressure. If the saphenofemoral junction is incompetent, it may be necessary first to prevent blood flowing back from the femoral vein by tying a tourniquet around the upper thigh.

CHRONIC VENOUS INSUFFICIENCY

Failure or inadequacy of the 'muscle pump' mechanism may also lead to chronic oedema of the legs and feet, with or without obvious varicose veins. The oedema is often relatively firm and pits only reluctantly on pressure; it is usually least apparent in the morning and gets worse as the day goes on.

VARICOSE ULCERATION AND ECZEMA

This may lead to skin necrosis and ulceration, most commonly at the ankle just above the malleoli. The skin is often dusky and indurated.

THROMBOPHLEBITIS

This commonly results either from local trauma or from an intravenous infusion but may occur spontaneously. There is local pain, redness and tenderness over the course of the vein.

DEEP VEIN THROMBOSIS

The characteristic clinical features of deep vein thrombosis in the leg are pain, swelling and occasionally redness. The leg may be swollen (compare it with the other one) and there is often dilatation of the superficial veins and a warm skin as a result of blood flow diversion from the deep to the superficial veins. Pain in the calf can sometimes be produced by dorsiflexing the foot but this can sometimes cause a detachment thrombus.

Clinically, pulmonary embolism may present in three ways: pulmonary infarction, acute massive pulmonary embolus and chronic thromboembolic pulmonary hypertension.

 Differential diagnosis
Deep vein thrombosis

Pain and swelling in the leg may be caused by:
- deep vein thrombosis
- ruptured head of gastrocnemius muscle
- ruptured osteoarthritic cyst (Baker's cyst) of knee joint
- anterior compartment syndrome

ACUTE PULMONARY INFARCTION

The clinical presentation is with the relatively sudden onset of pleuritic chest pain. The patient may be moderately breathless but is seldom hypotensive. Arterial blood gas measurements often show marked hypoxaemia, but the partial pressure of carbon dioxide is normal.

ACUTE MASSIVE PULMONARY EMBOLISM

This is most common in postoperative patients. The patient suddenly becomes extremely short of breath, severely hypotensive and may not be able to sit upright. The jugular veins are markedly distended and the liver may be enlarged. There may be a third sound, best heard to the left of the sternum. The chest radiograph is usually unhelpful but the ECG shows characteristic features of acute right ventricular strain.

CHRONIC PULMONARY HYPERTENSION

Chronic thromboembolic pulmonary hypertension is a result of multiple pulmonary emboli over a period of time. The clinical features are those of chronic pulmonary hypertension.

Infective endocarditis

ACUTE ENDOCARDITIS

Acute endocarditis is the result of infection of a normal or abnormal heart with a virulent organism such as *Staphylococcus aureus* or *Streptococcus pneumoniae*. The patient is nearly always severely ill with a fever and marked systemic symptoms. One of the characteristic clinical findings is that heart murmurs develop or change rapidly as the destructive process goes on. There may also be systemic emboli. There may be finger clubbing and splinter haemorrhages but often they do not have time to develop.

SUBACUTE ENDOCARDITIS

Subacute endocarditis may result either from infection of a diseased heart valve or septal defect with an indolent organism, such as *Streptococcus sanguis*, or from the partial treatment of acute endocarditis with inadequate doses of antibiotics. The time course of the illness is much more insidious. Patients present with unexplained fever, excessive tiredness or with the consequences of valve destruction or systemic embolisation. There is nearly always a heart murmur: the combination of fever and a heart murmur should always lead to suspicion of endocarditis. Finger clubbing and splinter haemorrhages are common. There is often splenomegaly. There may be localised subconjunctival haemorrhages, tender swellings (Osler's nodes) in the finger pulps and haemorrhagic spots (Roth spots) in the retina.

Myocarditis

Clinically, this may present with heart failure or an arrhythmia. There may be cardiac dilatation, a third heart sound or a systolic murmur from 'functional' mitral incompetence resulting from dilatation of the ventricle.

Cardiomyopathy

Cardiomyopathy is a general term meaning 'heart muscle disease'.

HYPERTROPHIC CARDIOMYOPATHY

The clinical features of hypertrophic obstructive cardiomyopathy are summarised in Figure 6.13.

DILATED CARDIOMYOPATHY

Dilated cardiomyopathy is characterised by a global impairment of left ventricular function, leading to progressive dilatation of the ventricles. Clinical presentation is usually with heart failure. There is a displaced apex beat, a gallop rhythm and possibly secondary mitral or tricuspid regurgitation.

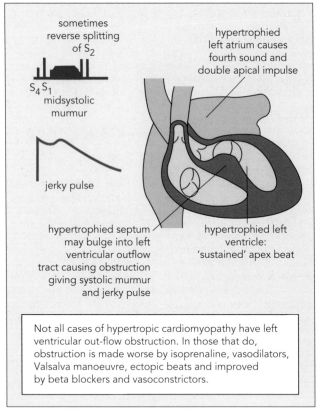

sometimes
reverse splitting
of S_2

hypertrophied
left atrium causes
fourth sound and
double apical impulse

S_4 S_1
midsystolic
murmur

jerky pulse

hypertrophied septum
may bulge into left
ventricular outflow
tract causing obstruction
giving systolic murmur
and jerky pulse

hypertrophied left
ventricle:
'sustained' apex beat

Not all cases of hypertropic cardiomyopathy have left
ventricular out-flow obstruction. In those that do,
obstruction is made worse by isoprenaline, vasodilators,
Valsalva manoeuvre, ectopic beats and improved
by beta blockers and vasoconstrictors.

Fig. 6.13 Findings in hypertrophic cardiomyopathy.

RESTRICTIVE CARDIOMYOPATHY
This is a rare condition in Western countries. The clinical presentation
mimics constrictive pericarditis.

Acute rheumatic fever

Clinically, acute rheumatic fever presents in children or young adults,
either with an acute, migratory (i.e. flitting from joint to joint)
polyarthritis or with chorea.

Cardiac involvement is usually signalled by the development of a
murmur: either a pansystolic murmur of mitral regurgitation or a soft
mid-diastolic murmur that resembles that of mitral stenosis. The latter
is called a Carey Coombs murmur. There is commonly a skin rash,

which again is often fleeting and variable. Rheumatic nodules are not seen in all cases but are virtually pathognomonic; they consist of firm subcutaneous nodules, often on the extensor surfaces of knees and elbows.

Pericardial disease

ACUTE PERICARDITIS

The most characteristic physical finding is the pericardial rub. This has a distinct scratchy quality. Pericardial rubs are often best heard if the patient is made to sit up, lean forward and breathe out fully. It is characteristic of a pericardial rub in that it comes and goes over a period of a few hours. Patients with acute pericarditis are often pyrexic and may feel systemically unwell.

PERICARDIAL EFFUSION

The patient is often very ill, hypotensive and peripherally constricted. There may be pulsus paradoxus. The jugular venous pressure is very high but this may be hard to see because the patient may be too hypotensive to sit upright. The best way of confirming the diagnosis

Differential diagnosis
Pericardial effusion

Infection
- Viral pericarditis
- Bacterial pericarditis (streptococcus)
- Tuberculous pericarditis

Myocardial infarction
- Peri-infarct pericarditis
- Cardiac rupture
- Dressler's syndrome

Malignant pericarditis
- Secondary (common) or primary (rare) tumours
- Leukaemia

Autoallergic
- Acute rheumatic fever
- Rheumatoid arthritis

Other
- Myxoedema
- Trauma (stab wounds)
- After cardiac surgery

is by bedside echocardiography, which can be followed immediately by pericardiocentesis.

The chronic pericardial effusion may be picked up by accident or (more commonly) it presents as chronic predominantly right-sided cardiac failure, often with very marked peripheral oedema and perhaps ascites. The jugular venous pressure is usually markedly elevated. There may be a paradoxical pulse but it is often less prominent than in acute cardiac tamponade.

CHRONIC CONSTRICTIVE PERICARDITIS

Chronic as opposed to acute inflammation of the pericardium may led to a thickened fibrotic pericardial membrane that, as a long-term result of scarring, constricts and compresses the heart.

The clinical features of chronic constrictive pericarditis are similar to those of chronic pericardial effusion. There tends to be predominantly right-sided heart failure, often with massive oedema. The jugular venous pressure is elevated and often has a characteristic pulse wave-form, with a very rapid dip in the pulse as the tricuspid valve opens, followed by an equally abrupt termination as filling of the ventricle is curtailed.

Examination of elderly people
Cardiovascular examination

- General approach and techniques unaltered
- Some stress tests may be impractical but there are alternatives
- Likely to be multisystem disease
- Common problems are hypertension, ischaemic heart disease and peripheral vascular disease
- Ischaemic heart disease may be asymptomatic
- Acute myocardial infarction may be 'silent'
- Ankle swelling usually clue to venous insufficiency not heart failure
- Aortic stenosis is common and difficult to diagnose but worth treating if severe
- Cardiac arrhythmias are common and do not generally require investigation unless symptomatic
- Causes of dizziness or transient loss of consciousness include postural hypotension (often drug induced), vertebrobasilar insufficiency, arrhythmias (especially bradycardia)
- Multiple drug therapy may be the cause of the problem – nonsteroidals cause fluid retention and hypertension

Review
Framework for routine examination of the cardiovascular system

1. While taking the history, watch the patient's face for features of anxiety, distress, breathlessness or features of specific diseases
2. Take the patient's hand and assess warmth, sweating and peripheral cyanosis; examine the nails for clubbing or splinter haemorrhages
3. Palpate the radial pulse and assess the rate and rhythm
4. Locate and palpate the brachial pulse and assess its character. Measure the blood pressure. If there is any suspicion of a problem with the aortic arch, compare pulses in both arms
5. With the patient lying supine at 45°, assess the jugular venous pressure and the jugular venous pulse form
6. Take an opportunity for a closer look at the face, the conjunctivae, the tongue and the inside of the mouth
7. Palpate the carotid pulse and assess its character
8. With the patient's chest exposed, inspect the precordium and assess the breathing pattern and the presence of any abnormal pulsation
9. Palpate the precordium, locate the apex beat and assess its character. Assess the feel of the rest of the precordium and the presence of any abnormal vibrations or thrills
10. Listen with the stethoscope and assess heart sounds and murmurs. If appropriate, listen over the carotid artery for radiating murmurs or bruits
11. Percuss and auscultate the chest both front and back looking for pleural effusions. Listen for crepitations at the lung bases
12. Lie the patient flat and palpate the abdomen, feeling in particular for the liver and any dilatation of the abdominal aorta
13. Assess the femoral pulses and the popliteal and foot pulses. Look for ankle or sacral oedema
14. If appropriate, assess the patient's exercise tolerance by taking the patient for a short walk
15. Test the urine

7.
The Abdomen

SYMPTOMS OF ABDOMINAL DISORDERS

Gastrointestinal diseases

DYSPHAGIA

Dysphagia caused by a carcinoma usually progresses rapidly over 6–10 weeks and is worse for solids than liquids. Profound weight loss results from reduced food intake and the wasting effect of the cancer.

Patients with a benign 'peptic' stricture often have a long history of heartburn, a slower rate of progression and less marked weight loss. In dysmotility syndromes the dysphagia often varies in intensity and is not accompanied by profound weight loss. Solids and fluids may be equally difficult to swallow. When dysphagia is caused by disease of the swallowing centre in the brainstem the symptom is accompanied by coughing and spluttering.

Questions to ask
Dysphagia

- At what level does food stick?
- Has the symptom developed over weeks, months or longer?
- Is the dysphagia intermittent or progressive?
- Are both food and drink equally difficult to swallow?
- Is there a history of reflux symptoms?

Differential diagnosis
Dysphagia

- Benign oesophageal stricture
- Carcinoma of the oesophagus
- Oesophageal motor disorders
- Systemic sclerosis
- Old age (presbyoesophagus)
- Bulbar and pseudobulbar palsy

HEARTBURN

The pain is a scalding or burning sensation behind the sternum and radiates towards the throat. An acid taste may develop in the mouth and reflex salivation may cause it to fill with saliva (water brash).

A common cause of heartburn is a hiatus hernia. Heartburn is often provoked by postures that raise intra-abdominal pressure, such as stooping, bending or lying down.

PAIN ON SWALLOWING (ODYNOPHAGIA)

The symptoms suggest deep inflammation or ulceration of the oesophageal wall or intense spasm of the oesophagus.

LOSS OF APPETITE (ANOREXIA)

A nonspecific symptom that commonly accompanies both acute and chronic ill health; return of appetite usually heralds recovery.

Profound anorexia occurs in anorexia nervosa, a psychiatric disorder occurring mainly in young women. Anorexia in these patients results in marked weight loss, malnutrition and cessation of menstruation (amenorrhoea). Suspect anorexia nervosa in teenagers and young adults, otherwise healthy, who present with an eating disorder associated with depression, vomiting or purgative abuse.

WEIGHT LOSS

Weight loss may be caused by inappropriate wastage of calories due to steatorrhoea, thyrotoxicosis or diabetes mellitus. Marked weight loss accompanies serious diseases such as chronic pancreatitis, advanced malignancy, chronic infections and failure of the major organs.

Questions to ask
Weight loss

- Is your appetite normal, increased or decreased?
- Over what time span has the weight been lost?
- Do you enjoy your meals?
- Describe your usual breakfast, lunch and supper
- Is the weight loss associated with nausea, vomiting or abdominal pain?
- Are your motions normal in colour and consistency?
- Has there been a fever?
- Do you pass excessive volumes of urine?
- Have you noticed a recent change in weather tolerance?

DYSPEPSIA AND INDIGESTION

This term applies to a sensation of pain, discomfort or fullness in the epigastrium, often accompanied by belching, nausea and early satiety.

Risk factors
Dyspepsia

- Cigarette smoking
- Alcohol
- Aspirin
- Nonsteroidal anti-inflammatory drugs (NSAIDs)
- Corticoteroids and NSAIDs
- Oral bisphosphonates
- *Helicobacter pylori* infection

Differential diagnosis
Dyspepsia

- Nonulcer dyspepsia
- Peptic ulcer disease
- Gastritis
- Gallstones
- Chronic pancreatitis

NAUSEA

Nausea usually comes in waves and is often associated with belching. The symptom may be provoked by unpleasant sights, smells and tastes or by abnormal stimulation or the inner ear labyrinths (motion sickness). It is a characteristic of the prodromal phase of viral hepatitis and often accompanies biliary disease. Drugs causing gastric irritation (e.g. nonsteroidal analgesics) or those stimulating the vomiting centre (e.g. digoxin) cause nausea. Early morning nausea commonly occurs during the first trimester of pregnancy.

VOMITING AND HAEMATEMESIS

Vomiting may occur in diseases of the gastrointestinal and biliary tracts, as well as in a variety of systemic and metabolic disorders. It may also be the presenting symptom of psychological disorders such as anorexia nervosa, bulimia and fear. Try to establish whether the vomit is bile-stained because this indicates patency between the stomach and duodenum. The presence of undigested food and a lack of bile suggest pyloric obstruction. Early morning vomiting is characteristic of alcoholism.

Vomiting blood (haematemesis) indicates bleeding from the oesophagus, stomach or duodenum. If the bleeding is brisk the vomit may be heavily bloodstained but if bleeding is slower or vomiting delayed, gastric acid reacts with haemoglobin, turning it a dark brown or 'coffee-ground' colour. If the bleeding is preceded by repeated bouts

Differential diagnosis
Gastrointestinal bleeding

Cause	Frequency
Gastric ulcer	30
Duodenal ulcer	21
Gastritis or erosions	9
Oesophagitis or oesophageal ulcer	8
Duodenitis	4
Varices	3
Tumours	2
Mallory–Weiss tear	1
Others	22

Emergency
Assessment of patient presenting with haematemesis and melena

- Pulse rate
- Respiratory rate
- Recumbent blood pressure
- Evidence of postural hypotension and reduced capillary filling time
- Hydration (dry tongue, sunken eyes, reduced skin turgor)
- Pallor (caused by shock and peripheral vasoconstriction or anaemia)
- Urine output
- Stigmata of liver disease (flap, jaundice, spider naevi)

of retching or vomiting, consider as the cause a Mallory–Weiss tear, which results from mechanical disruption of the mucosa at the gastro-oesophageal junction. Enquire about ingestion of alcohol or other gastric irritants (e.g. aspirin). If there is evidence of coincident liver disease, consider oesophageal varices to be the cause of bleeding. Weight loss may suggest bleeding from a gastric cancer, and a history of epigastric pain or heartburn suggests bleeding from a peptic ulcer or ulcerated oesophagus.

ABDOMINAL PAIN
When taking a history of abdominal pain, aim to distinguish between visceral, parietal and referred pain.

? Questions to ask
Abdominal pain

- Describe the position, character and radiation of the pain
- Has the pain been present for hours, days, weeks, months or years?
- Is the pain constant or intermittent?
- Have you noticed specific aggravating or relieving factors?
- Is the pain affected by eating or defecation?
- Does the pain awake you from sleep?
- Is there associated nausea or vomiting?
- Has there been associated weight loss?
- Is there a history of ulcerogenic drugs?
- Has there been a change in bowel habit?

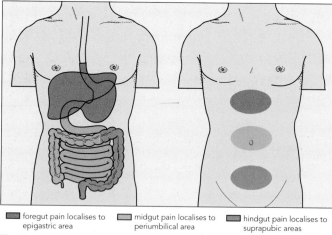

▬ foregut pain localises to epigastric area	▭ midgut pain localises to periumbilical area	▬ hindgut pain localises to suprapubic areas

Fig. 7.1 Perception of visceral pain is localised to the epigastric, umbilical or suprapubic region according to the embryological origin of the diseased organ.

Visceral pain is caused by stretching or inflammation of a hollow muscular organ (gut, gallbladder, bile duct, ureters, uterus). It is perceived near the midline, irrespective of the location of the organ (Fig. 7.1). Visceral pain may also radiate to specific sites and this helps to establish its origin (Fig. 7.2).

Colic, signifies obstruction of a hollow, muscular organ, such as the intestine, gallbladder, bile duct or ureter, and consists of recurring

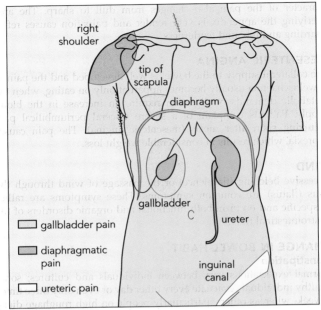

Fig. 7.2 Characteristic radiation of pain from the gallbladder, diaphragm and ureters. The pain is not always felt in the organ concerned.

bouts of intense, cramping pain. When the smaller organs such as the gallbladder, bile duct or ureters are acutely obstructed by a stone, the cyclical nature of colic soon gives way to a continuous visceral pain caused by the inflammatory effect of the impacted stone or secondary infection. Movement does not aggravate visceral pain, so the patient may writhe or double up in response to it.

Pain arising from the parietal peritoneum is well localised to the area immediately overlying the area of inflammation or irritation. The patient lies as still as possible. Palpation over the area is extremely painful, with the overlying muscles contracting to protect the peritoneum (guarding). When the pressure of the examining hand is suddenly released, the pain is further aggravated and the patient winces. This sign is known as 'rebound tenderness'.

Abdominal pain may progress from a visceral sensation to a parietal pain. Acute appendicitis provides an excellent example of this transition. When this midgut structure becomes inflamed and obstructed, a dull pain localises to the periumbilical area. As the inflammation to the parietal peritoneum, the pain appears to shift to the right iliac fossa, where it localises over McBurney's point. The character of the pain also changes from dull to sharp. The area overlying the appendix is very tender and palpation causes reflex guarding and rebound tenderness.

MESENTERIC ANGINA

The collateral supply to the bowel is well developed and the pain of bowel ischaemia usually becomes apparent only on eating, when the metabolic demands of digestion require an increase in the blood supply. Patients complain of a severe visceral periumbilical pain occurring soon after meals (mesenteric angina). The pain causes anorexia, which results in considerable weight loss.

WIND

Excessive belching (flatulence) or the passage of wind through the anus (flatus) are common symptoms. These symptoms are rather unspecific and occur in both functional and organic disorders of the gastrointestinal tract.

CHANGE IN BOWEL HABIT
Constipation

Normal expectations vary between individuals and cultures; some healthy individuals evacuate every other day or even only three times a week, whereas others, particularly people on high roughage diets, expect up to three bulky bowel actions daily. Constipation is described more precisely as a disorder of bowel habit characterised by straining and the infrequent passage of small, hard stools. Patients often complain that they are left with a sense of incomplete evacuation (tenesmus).

When constipation presents as a recent change, and especially if it is associated with colic, suspect an organic cause such as malignancy

Differential diagnosis
Constipation

- Low-residue diet
- Motility disorder (functional bowel disease)
- Physical immobility
- Drugs (especially opiates and antidepressants)
- Depression and dementia
- Organic disease
  - colon cancer
  - diverticular stricture
  - Crohn's stricture
  - hypothyroidism
  - electrolyte imbalance

or stricture formation. Enquire about constipating drugs (e.g. codeine-containing analgesics) and rectal bleeding, an alarm symptom that raises the suspicion of cancer. Consider hypothyroidism or electrolyte abnormalities. Anal pain caused by a fissure or a thrombosed pile may cause profound constipation because of the patient's fear of pain at stool.

Constipation caused by chronic partial obstruction may be punctuated by periods of loose or watery stool. This 'spurious diarrhoea' occurs in elderly patients with faecal impaction and also when colon cancer causes a partial obstruction. The proximal bowel dilates and fills with liquid, which then seeps around the obstruction, presenting as liquid diarrhoea.

Diarrhoea

Diarrhoea implies increased stool volume and frequency and a change in consistency from formed to semiformed, semiliquid or liquid. Functional diarrhoea caused by anxiety, stress or the irritable bowel syndrome does not wake the patient from sleep. Recent travel abroad, eating out or an outbreak among people living in close proximity suggests an infective cause.

Enquire about colour; in fat malabsorption, the stool is pale, malodorous, poorly formed and difficult to flush. When a cause is not readily apparent, consider laxative abuse and recent broad-spectrum antibiotic treatment.

Questions to ask
Diarrhoea

- What is the normal stool frequency?
- How many stools daily?
- How long have you had diarrhoea?
- Are you awoken from sleep to open the bowels?
- What is the colour and consistency of stools?
- Are blood and mucus present?
- Any travel abroad or contact with diarrhoea?
- Is there associated nausea, vomiting, weight loss or pain?
- Any purgative abuse?
- Any antibiotics?

Rectal bleeding

Bright-red rectal bleeding usually arises from the sigmoid colon or rectum and more proximal colonic bleeding is often a darker red or maroon colour. In haemorrhoidal bleeding the blood may be most noticeable on the toilet paper. Colon cancer and polyps often present with intermittent rectal bleeding, whereas patients with inflammatory bowel disease pass blood, often mixed with mucus, with each stool. Torrential haemorrhage may occur from diverticular disease and marked bleeding may occur in mesenteric vascular disease. Microscopic blood loss (occult bleeding) usually presents with symptoms of anaemia. Always consider a diagnosis of gastric, caecal or colon cancer in older patients with unexplained iron deficiency anaemia.

The passage of sticky, black stools with the consistency of tar (melaena) usually indicates bleeding from the oesophagus, stomach or duodenum. Treatment with iron and certain drugs (e.g. bismuth-containing preparations) also blackens the stool and must be distinguished from melaena.

Liver disease

Liver cell damage and obstruction of the bile duct both have numerous clinical consequences, the most striking of which are jaundice, pale stools and darkening of the urine.

In patients with portal hypertension, portal blood bypasses the liver (portosystemic shunting), and the brain is exposed to gut-derived products which depress brain function, causing hepatic encephalopathy.

A further clinical consequence of portal hypertension is fluid retention in the abdominal cavity (ascites).

LIVER CELL DAMAGE

Symptoms of liver damage are not very specific and include malaise, fatigue, anorexia and nausea. Viral hepatitis is preceded by prodromes such as fatigue, nausea and a profound distaste for alcohol and cigarettes. Before the onset of jaundice the patient may notice darkening of the urine and lightening of stool colour.

Enquire about the principal causes of liver damage. Calculate the number of units (or grams) of alcohol consumed in a week. Ask about foreign travel, intravenous drug abuse or exposure to blood products,

Risk factors
Factors predisposing to hepatitis B

- Intravenous drug abuse
- Exposure to contaminated blood or blood products
- Reuse of hypodermic needles
- Unprotected sex
- Needle-stick injury from infected individual
- Vertical transmission from mother to newborn

and establish the patient's sexual orientation. Enquire about drugs that may cause liver damage and ask about a family history of liver disease.

If encephalopathy occurs, the sleep pattern may be reversed and the patient may undergo a change in personality.

Questions to ask
Jaundice

- Have you travelled to areas where hepatitis A is endemic?
- Is there a history of alcohol or intravenous drug abuse?
- Have you ever had a blood transfusion?
- Have you had contact with jaundiced patients?
- Have you experienced skin itching?
- What medication has been used recently (including nonprescription drugs)?
- Have you had occupational contact with hepatotoxins?
- Is there pain and weight loss?
  What colour are the stools and urine?
- Is there a family history of liver disease?

Differential diagnosis
Jaundice

Prehepatic or unconjugated hyperbilirubinaemia
- Haemolytic anaemias
- Gilbert's syndrome

Hepatocellular disease
- Viral hepatitis (types A, B, C, D and E)
- Alcoholic hepatitis
- Autoimmune hepatitis (lupoid)
- Drug hepatitis (halothane, paracetamol)
- Decompensated cirrhosis

Intrahepatic cholestasis
- Drugs (phenothiazines)
- Primary biliary cirrhosis
- Primary sclerosing cholangitis

Extrahepatic cholestasis
- Bile duct stricture (benign and malignant)
- Common duct stone
- Cancer of the head of the pancreas

Biliary obstruction

The principal symptom is itching (pruritus) and this may occur long before the patient becomes jaundiced. As with viral hepatitis, lightening of the stools and darkening of the urine often precedes jaundice. Severe epigastric and right hypochondrial pain accompanied by fever and jaundice suggests impaction of a gallstone in the common bile duct, whereas 'painless' jaundice suggests either a more chronic obstruction of the common bile duct (e.g. cancer of either the bile duct or head of the pancreas) or damage to the intrahepatic biliary tree (e.g. primary biliary cirrhosis, sclerosing cholangitis, drugs).

Pancreatic disease

Acute pancreatitis presents with the onset of upper abdominal pain that is most prominent in the epigastrium and left upper quadrant. The pain may radiate through to the back, with its intensity varying from mild to severe. Some relief may be obtained by sitting forward. Ask about alcohol intake and drugs (e.g. azathioprine, furosemide (frusemide), corticoids) and consider underlying gallstones, which may precipitate acute pancreatitis.

Recurrent attacks of acute pancreatitis may result in chronic pancreatitis. This is often characterised by persistent, severe upper abdominal pain that may radiate circumferentially to the back. Progressive loss of exocrine function eventually leads to steatorrhoea and weight loss.

Kidney and bladder disease

FREQUENCY AND URGENCY

Frequency refers to the desire to pass urine more often than normal. Urgency may accompany frequency (i.e. a strong urge to urinate even though only small amounts of urine are present in the bladder).

 Symptoms and signs
Some renal symptoms and their causes

Frequency
- Irritable bladder
  - infection, inflammation, chemical irritation
- Reduced compliance
  - fibrosis, tumour infiltration
- Bladder outlet obstruction
  - in prostatism, detrusor failure may limit the volume voided

Symptoms and signs
Some renal symptoms and their causes – *(cont'd)*

Polyuria
- Ingestion of large volumes of water, beverages or alcohol
- Chronic renal failure (loss of concentrating power)
- Diabetes mellitus (osmotic effect of glucose in urine)
- Diabetes insipidus (caused by a lack of ADH or tubules insensitive to circulating ADH)
- Diuretic treatment

Dysuria
- Bacterial infection of the bladder (cystitis)
- Inflammation of the urethra (urethritis)
- Infection or inflammation of the prostate (prostatitis)

Incontinence
- Sphincter damage or weakness after childbirth
- Sphincter weakness in old age
- Prostate cancer
- Benign prostatic hypertrophy
- Spinal cord disease, paraplegia

Oliguria or anuria
- Hypovolaemia (dehydration or shock)
- Acute renal failure caused by acute glomerulonephritis
- Bilateral ureteric obstruction (retroperitoneal fibrosis)
- Detrusor muscle failure (bladder outlet obstruction or neurological disease)

NOCTURIA

This may occur in patients with daytime frequency or individuals producing excessive quantities of urine (polyuria). Incomplete bladder voiding caused by prostatism often presents with nocturia.

INCONTINENCE

If the symptom is provoked by increased intra-abdominal pressure (coughing, sneezing or laughing), it is referred to as 'stress incontinence'.

Diseases causing excessive bladder filling (e.g. bladder outlet obstruction) may cause 'overflow incontinence' which reflects spill-over from an overfilled, hypotonic bladder.

HESITANCY

Hesitancy is a delay between attempting to initiate urination and the actual flow of urine. It is a characteristic sign of bladder outlet obstruction (e.g. as a result of prostatic hypertrophy).

OLIGURIA AND ANURIA

The term oliguria is used if less than 500 ml of urine is passed over 24 h.

PAIN

Infection of the kidneys (pyelonephritis) causes pain and tenderness in the renal angles, usually associated with fever. Obstruction of the ureters by stones, sloughed papillae or blood may cause intense pain in the renal angle. This pain may radiate towards the groins and, in men, into the testes. Renal 'colic' caused by stones in the ureters is extremely painful, often causing the patient to double-up or roll around. Bladder pain may occur in severe cystitis. The pain is localised to the suprapubic region and associated with urgency and frequency.

DYSURIA

Dysuria describes a stinging or burning sensation that occurs when passing urine. The most common cause of dysuria is cystitis.

HAEMATURIA

Blood in urine may be obvious, associated with a cloudy colour or only apparent on chemical testing (microscopic haematuria).

 Differential diagnosis
Haematuria

Painful
- Kidney stones
- Urinary tract infection
- Papillary necrosis

Painless
- Infection
- Cancer of the urinary tract
- Acute glomerulonephritis
- Contamination during menstruation

EXAMINATION OF THE ABDOMEN

For descriptive purposes the anterior abdominal wall may be divided into four quadrants (Fig. 7.3). The abdomen may also be divided into nine segments resembling a 'noughts and crosses' matrix.

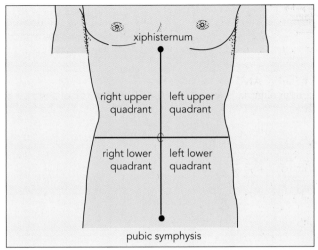

Fig. 7.3 The quadrants of the anterior abdominal wall.

Inspection of the abdomen

CONTOURS

The normal abdomen is concave and symmetrical and moves gently with respiration. In thin individuals you may notice the pulsation of the abdominal aorta in the midline above the umbilicus.

Fluid gravitates towards the flanks, causing the loins to bulge, and the umbilicus may become everted. Suprapubic fullness may reflect an enlarged uterus (pregnancy or fibroids), ovaries (cysts or carcinoma) or a full bladder. The periodic rippling movement of bowel peristalsis may be observed in intestinal obstruction.

Surgical scars are potential points of weakness in the abdominal wall and incisional herniae may develop under the scar.

SKIN

After childbirth many women are left with tell-tale stretch lines (striae gravidarum). In Cushing's syndrome purplish striae appear on the abdominal wall even in the absence of a pregnancy. In acute haemorrhagic pancreatitis, there may be a bluish discoloration of either the flanks (Grey Turner's sign) or the periumbilical area (Cullen's sign), which results from seepage of bloodstained ascitic fluid along the fascial planes and into the subcutaneous tissue.

Look for veins coursing over the abdominal wall. The direction of flow helps distinguish normal from abnormal flow patterns (Fig. 7.4).

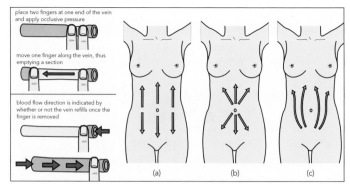

Fig. 7.4 Determining the direction of blood flow in abdominal veins. (a) Normal blood flow pattern and those characteristic of (b) portal hypertension and (c) obstruction of the inferior vena cava.

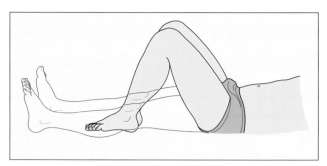

Fig. 7.5 Palpation of the abdomen may be aided if the patient is asked to flex the hips. This helps to relax the anterior abdominal wall.

Palpation of the abdomen

If the patient is not relaxed, ask the patient to bend the knees and flex the hips (Fig. 7.5). A single-handed technique may be used but you may prefer to use both hands, the upper hand applying pressure, while the lower hand concentrates on feeling.

LIGHT PALPATION

Ask the patient to localise any areas of pain or tenderness. Begin the examination in the segment furthest from the discomfort. Start light palpation by gently pressing your fingers into each of the nine segments, sustaining the light pressure for a few seconds while gently exploring each area with the fingertips.

In peritonitis, the patient flinches on even the lightest palpation and there is reflex rigidity, guarding and rebound tenderness.

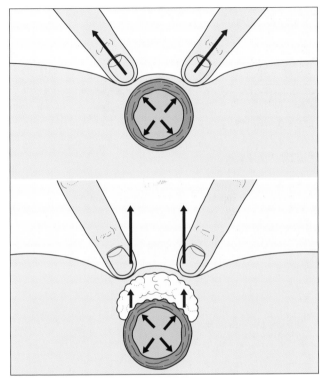

Fig. 7.6 Palpating the aorta. The direction of the pulsation indicates whether it arises directly from the aorta (above) or is transmitted by a mass overlying the tissues (below).

DEEP PALPATION

In thin individuals, the descending and sigmoid colon may be felt as an elongated tubular structure in the left loin and lower quadrant. The sigmoid is mobile and can readily be rolled under the fingers. The colon can usually be distinguished from other structures because of its firm stool content. It has a putty-like consistency and can be indented with the fingertips. The 'mass' also becomes less obvious after the passage of stool. In thin individuals, the abdominal aorta may be felt as a discrete pulsatile structure in the midline, above the umbilicus.

A large pulsatile structure in the midline above the umbilicus indicates an aortic aneurysm or a transmitted impulse to a mass overlying the aorta. These can usually be distinguished using the index finger of either hand to sense whether the movement is pulsatile or transmitted (Fig. 7.6).

PALPATION OF THE ORGANS
Palpating the liver

Use either the fingertips or the radial side of the index finger to explore for the liver edge under the costal margin. Point the ends of the index, middle and ring fingers in an upward position, facing the liver edge, at a point midway between the costal margin and iliac crests, lateral to the rectus muscle. Press the fingertips inwards and upwards and hold this position while the patient takes a deep inspiration. As the fingers drift upwards, feel for the liver edge slipping under them as the organ descends. If no edge is felt, repeat the manoeuvre in a stepwise fashion, each time moving the starting position a little closer to the costal margin.

It is useful to percuss for the lower liver edge. With the long axis of your middle finger positioned parallel to the right costal margin, percuss from the point where you started palpating for the liver. This point normally overlies bowel and should sound resonant. Repeat the percussion in a stepwise manner until the note becomes duller.

Find the position of the upper margin of the liver. Percuss the third space and then percuss each succeeding interspace until you detect the transition from resonance to dullness. Measure the liver span in the midclavicular line; in women this should measure 8–10 cm and in men, 10–12 cm.

Differential diagnosis
Hepatomegaly

- Macronodular cirrhosis
- Neoplastic disease (primary and secondary cancer, myeloproliferative disorders)
- Infections (viral hepatitis, tuberculosis, hydatid disease)
- Infiltrations (iron, fat, amyloid, Gaucher's disease)

General signs of liver disease

Look for jaundice in the sclerae.

Vascular spiders (spider naevi) consist of a central arteriole from which branch a series of smaller vessels. Spider naevi are found in the territory drained by the superior vena cava. The central arteriole can be occluded with a pencil tip and on release of the pressure the vessels rapidly refill from the centre.

The physical sign characteristic of hepatic encephalopathy is a 'flapping tremor'. Ask the patient to stretch out both arms and hyper-extend the wrists with the fingers held separated (Fig. 7.7). A coarse, involuntary flap occurs at the wrist and metacarpophalangeal joints.

Symptoms and signs
Signs of liver disease

General examination
- Nutrition status
- Pallor (blood loss)
- Jaundice
- Breath fetor of liver failure
- Xanthelasmata (chronic cholestasis)
- Parotid swelling (alcohol abuse)
- Bruising (clotting diathesis)
- Spider naevi
- Female distribution of body hair

Mental state
- Wernicke's or Korsakoff's psychosis
- Flapping tremor of hepatic encephalopathy
- Inability to copy a five-pointed star

Hands
- Leuconychia (hypoproteinaemia)
- Liver flap
- Palmar erythema
- Dupuytren's contractures
- Mild finger clubbing

Chest
- Gynaecomastia
- Right-sided pleural effusion

Abdomen
- Dilated veins
- Liver or spleen enlargement
- Ascites
- Testicular atrophy

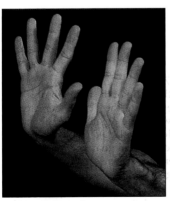

Fig. 7.7 To elicit a flapping tremor in hepatic encephalopathy, ask the patient to stretch out the arms with the hands extended at the wrist and metacarpophalangeal joints. This position is held for 20 seconds.

Symptoms and signs
Child-Pugh classification of severity of liver disease

Parameter	Points assigned		
	1	2	3
Ascites	Absent	Slight	Moderate
Albumin (g/l)	>35	28–35	<28
INR (clotting)	<1.7	1.8–2.3	>2.3
Encephalopathy	None	Grade 1–2	Grade 3–4

Score
- 5–6 = Grade A (well-compensated disease)
- 7–9 = Grade B (significant functional disturbance)
- 10–15 = Grade C (decompensated liver disease)

Prognosis (%)

	1 year	2 year
Grade A	100	85
Grade B	80	60
Grade C	45	35

Risk factors
Cirrhosis

- Alcoholism
- Chronic hepatitis B
- Chronic hepatitis C
- Chronic biliary disease (sclerosing cholangitis, primary biliary cirrhosis)
- Iron overload
- Autoimmune disease
- Copper overload

Palpating the gallbladder (Fig. 7.8)

This surface marking coincides with the tip of the right 9th rib.

Using gentle but firm pressure palpate the gallbladder area by pointing the tips of the fingers towards the organ while the patient inspires deeply. When the gallbladder is inflamed (cholecystitis), the most striking physical sign is tenderness and guarding over the gall-bladder region. The patient experiences intense pain, winces and interrupts the breath (Murphy's sign).

Palpating the spleen

Start the examination from the region of the umbilicus. Position the fingers of the right hand obliquely across the abdomen, with the

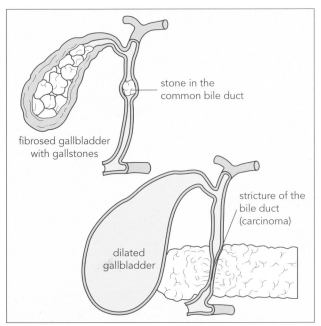

Fig. 7.8 If jaundice is caused by impaction of a gallstone in the bile duct, the fibrosed, stone-filled gallbladder does not dilate. However, if jaundice is caused by a bile duct stricture the healthy gallbladder dilates and can be palpated as a soft mass arising from behind the 9th right rib anteriorly.

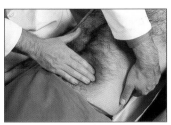

Fig. 7.9 When palpating the spleen use your left hand to support the ribcage posteriorly, while the fingertips of your right hand explore the leading edge of the organ.

fingertips pointing at the left costal margin and towards the axilla (Fig. 7.9). Using a moderate amount of pressure hold this steady while asking the patient to breathe in deeply. The notched leading edge of an enlarged spleen can be felt passing under the fingers and glancing off at the height of inspiration.

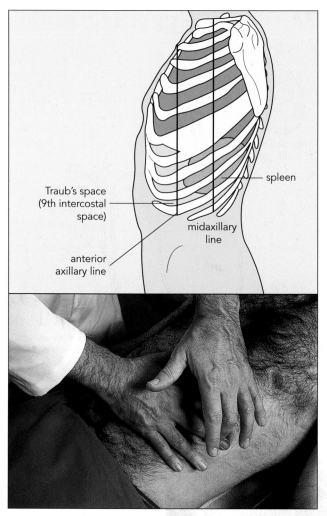

Fig. 7.10 After palpating for the spleen, percuss for the enlarged organ in the 9th intercostal space anterior to the anterior axillary line.

At this point in the examination percuss for splenic dullness. Percuss the 9th intercostal space anterior to the anterior axillary line (Traub's space) (Fig. 7.10). This space overlies bowel and is normally tympanitic, but as the solid spleen enlarges this area becomes less resonant, eventually sounding dull.

Examining the renal system

PALPATING THE KIDNEYS

The kidneys are retroperitoneal organs and deep bimanual palpation is required to explore for them. Tuck the palmar surfaces of the left hand posteriorly into the left flank and nestle the fingertips in the renal angle (Fig. 7.11a). Position the middle three fingers of the right hand below the left costal margin, lateral to the rectus muscle and at a point opposite the posterior hand (Fig. 7.11b). To examine the right kidney, tuck your left hand behind the right loin and position the fingers of your right hand below the right costal margin, lateral to rectus abdominis. Ask the patient to inspire deeply; press the fingers of both hands firmly together, attempting to capture the lower pole as it slips through the fingertips. This technique is known as ballotting the kidney.

The kidney may be tender, especially when acutely infected (pyelonephritis). This may be apparent on bimanual palpation, although a more specific sign is 'punch' tenderness over the renal angles.

 Symptoms and signs
Differentiation between splenomegaly and palpation of the left kidney

Kidney
- Moves late in inspiration
- Possible to get above upper pole
- Smooth shape
- Resonant to percussion

Enlarged spleen
- Moves early in inspiration
- Impossible to get above a spleen
- Notched leading edge
- Dull to percussion in Traub's space
- Enlarges towards umbilicus

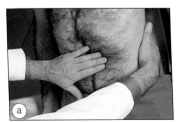 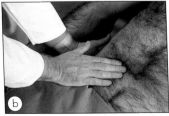

Fig. 7.11 Positioning the hands when palpating (a) the left and (b) the right kidney.

Palpating the aorta

The aorta can be palpated between the thumb and finger of one hand or by positioning the fingers of both hands on either side of the midline at a point midway between the xiphisternum and the umbilicus. Press the fingers posteriorly and slightly medially and feel for the pulsation of the abdominal aorta against your fingertips.

An abdominal aortic aneurysm may be felt as a large pulsatile mass above the level of the umbilicus.

Symptoms and signs
Signs of chronic renal failure

- Sallow complexion
- Anaemia (normocytic, normochromic)
- Uraemic fetor
- Deep acidotic breathing (Kussmaul respiration)
- Hypertension
- Mental clouding
- Uraemic encephalopathy (flapping tremor)
- Pleural and pericardial effusion
- Pericardial rub (pericarditis)
- Evidence of fluid overload or depletion
- Renal masses (polycystic kidneys)
- Large bladder (chronic bladder outlet obstruction)

Differential diagnosis
Chronic renal failure

- Chronic glomerulonephritis
- Systemic hypertension
- Diabetes mellitus with nephropathy
- Chronic obstructive uropathy
- Polycystic disease of the kidneys
- Analgesic nephropathy

Percussion of the abdomen

PERCUSSION TO DETECT ASCITES

The presence of ascites can be confirmed by altering the patient's posture and demonstrating a change in the position of the gas–fluid interface (Fig. 7.12).

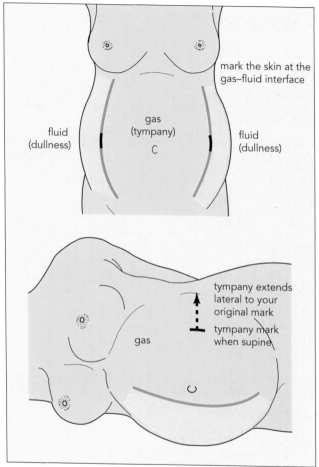

Fig. 7.12 To confirm the presence of ascites, roll the patient into the right lateral position because this causes fluid to settle in the dependent right flank, whereas gas-filled bowel floats above to fill the left flank. A shift in the positions of dullness and tympany indicates free fluid.

Repeat the percussion from the midline towards the left flank. The tympany should extend well lateral to the interface marked in supine examination.

PERCUSSION TO DETECT A DISTENDED BLADDER

A level of dullness above this landmark indicates the upper margin of a distended bladder or possibly enlargement of the uterus. An enlarged bladder is felt as a rounded fullness.

Auscultation of the abdomen

LISTENING FOR BOWEL SOUNDS

Place the diaphragm of the stethoscope on the midabdomen and listen for intermittent gurgling sounds (borborygma). These peristaltic sounds occur episodically at 5–10 s intervals, although longer silent periods may occur. Keep listening for approximately 30 s before concluding that bowel sound are reduced or absent.

The absence of any bowel sounds can indicate intestinal paralysis (paralytic ileus). In progressive bowel obstruction, large amounts of gas and fluid accumulate and the bowel sounds change in quality to a higher pitched 'tinkling'.

In pyloric obstruction, the stomach distends with gas and fluid; this can be detected by listening for 'succussion splash'. Shake the upper abdomen for the splashing sound characteristic of gastric outflow obstruction.

LISTENING FOR ARTERIAL BRUITS

Position the diaphragm of the stethoscope over the abdominal aorta. A systolic murmur (a bruit) indicates turbulent flow and suggests arteriosclerosis or an aneurysm.

Listen for renal arterial bruits at a point 2.5 cm above and lateral to the umbilicus. The presence of a renal bruit suggests congenital or arteriosclerotic renal artery stenosis or narrowing caused by fibromuscular hyperplasia.

EXAMINING THE GROINS

EXAMINING HERNIAE

An inguinal hernia usually presents as a lump in the groin so it is best to examine the hernia with the patient standing. Place two fingers on the mass and ascertain whether or not an impulse is transmitted to your fingertips when the patient coughs. Most herniae can be reduced manually. Once the hernia is fully reduced, occlude the internal ring with a finger pressing over the femoral point. Ask the patient to cough. An indirect inguinal hernia should not reappear until you release the occlusion of the internal ring.

A direct inguinal hernia develops through a weakness in the posterior wall of the inguinal canal. These herniae seldom force their way into the scrotum and, once reduced, their reappearance is not controlled by pressure over the internal ring.

When an inguinal hernia extends as far as the external ring it may be confused with a femoral hernia. An inguinal hernia lies above and medial to the tubercle, whereas a femoral hernia lies below and lateral.

EXAMINING THE ANUS, RECTUM AND PROSTATE

Rectum and anus

Lubricate your index finger with water-soluble gel and press the fingertip against the anal verge with the pulp facing the 6 o'clock position. Slip your finger into the anal canal and then insert it into the rectum, directing the tip posteriorly to follow the sacral curve. With your finger fully introduced, check on anal tone by asking the patient to squeeze your finger with the anal muscles. Then gently sweep the finger through 180° using the palmar surface of the finger to explore the posterior and posterolateral walls of the rectum. Rotate the finger round to the 12 o'clock position. The normal rectum feels uniformly smooth and pliable. In men, the prostate can be felt anteriorly and in women it may be possible to feel the cervix as well as a retroverted uterus.

Withdraw your finger from the rectum and anus and check the glove tip for stool. There may be melaena, blood or pus and you may notice the pale, greasy stools characteristic of malabsorption.

Prostate

The gland has a rubbery, smooth consistency and a shallow longitudinal groove separates the right and left lobes.

Palpation of the prostate aims to assess size, consistency, nodularity and tenderness. Benign hypertrophy of the prostate is smooth and symmetrical and the gland feels rubbery or slightly boggy. A cancerous prostate may feel asymmetric, with a stony hard consistency, and discrete nodules may be palpable. Marked prostatic tenderness suggests acute prostatitis, a prostatic abscess or inflammation of the seminal vesicles.

Examination of elderly people
Abdominal examination in elderly people

- On inspection of the abdomen there may be asymmetry caused by kyphoscoliosis of the spine
- Osteoporosis and deformity of the ribcage causes the costal margin to migrate towards the pelvis, making abdominal examination more difficult
- If the patient is hard of hearing or dyspraxic there may be difficulty in obtaining the cooperation needed to palpate the liver and spleen

Examination of elderly people
Abdominal examination in elderly people – *(cont'd)*

- Constipation in the elderly often manifests with the impression of a mass in the left lower quadrant (this can be reassessed after an enema to induce evacuation)
- An ectatic aorta is often palpable and scoliosis often displaces the aorta, giving a false impression of an aortic aneurysm
- Consider an aneurysm if the aorta is assessed to be greater than 5 cm in diameter at its widest (readily confirmed on ultrasound)
- Aortic bruits are more common in the elderly, reflecting atherosclerosis or aneurysm
- Leaking aneurysm may present as backache and rupture presents as an acute abdominal emergency with shock, abdominal distension, poor distal perfusion and asymmetrical pulses
- Benign or malignant prostatic hypertrophy in older men predisposes to bladder outlet obstruction, detrusor instability and failure, urinary retention and infection
- Acute urinary retention is a common cause of acute 'unexplained' confusion in the elderly: always examine for an enlarged bladder in elderly patients presenting with confusion, delirium, incontinence or fever
- Faecal incontinence may be associated with dementia, chronic constipation with overflow, laxative abuse and disordered sphincteric function
- A rectal examination and plain abdominal X-ray usually clarify faecal impaction in the elderly

Review
The abdominal examination

General examination
- Nutrition and hydration
- Peripheral oedema (hypoproteinaemia)
- Leuconychia or koilonychia
- Signs of liver disease

Inspection
- Shape and symmetry
- Scars and striae
- Abdominal wall veins and flow pattern

- Visible peristalsis
- Hernias (paraumbilical, inguinal)

Palpation (nine segments)
- Light palpation to assess tenderness
- Deeper palpation for masses
- Liver, spleen, kidneys
- Bladder, uterus, aorta

Review
The abdominal examination – *(cont'd)*

Percussion
- Upper and lower liver margins
- Spleen (Traub's space)
- Shifting dullness (ascites)
- Suprapubic dullness (bladder)

Auscultation
- Bowel sounds
- Aortic and renal bruits
- Hepatic and splenic rubs

Rectal examination
- Rectal mucosa
- Prostate, uterus

8.
Female Breasts and Genitalia

SYMPTOMS OF BREAST DISEASE

Pain

This dynamic response of the tissue to changes in hormones may cause breast pain and tenderness which fluctuates predictably with the menstrual cycle. A painful breast in the first few months of lactation is almost always due to a bacterial infection of the gland and is characterised by fever, redness and tenderness over the infected segment.

Discharge

Determine whether the fluid is clear, opalescent or bloodstained. After childbearing, some women continue to discharge a small secretion well after lactation has stopped. The inappropriate secretion of milk (galactorrhoea) is caused by a deranged prolactin physiology. A blood discharge should always alert you to the likelihood of an underlying breast cancer.

Breast lumps

A patient may present after discovering a breast lump by self-examination.

 Differential diagnosis
Breast lumps

Benign
- Fibroadenoma (mobile)
- Simple cyst
- Fat necrosis
- Fibroadenosis (tender 'lumpy' breasts)
- Abscess (painful and tender)

Malignant
- Glandular
- Areolar

EXAMINATION OF THE BREAST

Inspection

The patient should undress to the waist. Position yourself in front of the patient, who should be sitting comfortably with her arms at her side (Fig. 8.1). Ask the patient to raise her arms above her head and then press her hands against her hips. These movements tighten the suspensory ligaments, exaggerating the contours and highlighting any abnormality.

Symptoms and signs
Breast examination

Inspection
- Symmetry and contour
- Venous pattern of skin
- Nipples (asymmetry, inversion)
- Areola (chloasma, skin ulceration, thickening)

Breast palpation
- Texture
- Symmetry

- Tenderness
- Masses (mobility, size)
- Tail of Spence

Lymph node palpation
- Axillary nodes (five groups)
- Contralateral axillary nodes
- Infraclavicular and supraclavicular nodes

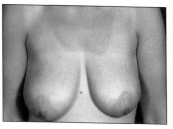

Fig. 8.1 Initially, inspect the breast from the front with the patient sitting with her arms comfortably resting at her sides.

ABNORMALITIES ON INSPECTION

You may be struck by an obvious lump, retraction or gross deviation of a nipple, prominent veins or oedema of the skin with dimpling like an orange skin (peau d'orange). Abnormal reddening, thickening or ulceration of the areola should alert you to the possibility of Paget's disease of the breast, a specialised form of breast cancer.

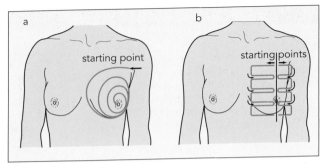

Fig. 8.2 Trace a systematic path either by following a concentric circular pattern (a) or examining each half of the breast sequentially from above down (b).

Breast palpation

Examine each breast by following a concentric or parallel trail that creates a systematic path that always begins and ends at a constant spot (Fig. 8.2). A comparison of the two breasts may help you to judge whether an area is abnormal or not.

To examine the axillary tail of Spence, ask the patient to rest her arms above her head. Feel the tail between your thumb and fingers as it extends from the upper outer quadrant towards the axilla. If you feel a breast lump, examine the mass between your fingers and assess its size, consistency, mobility and whether or not there is any tenderness.

Nipple palpation

Hold the nipple between thumb and fingers and gently compress and attempt to express any discharge. If fluid appears, note its colour, prepare a smear for cytology and send a swab for microbiology.

Lymph node palpation

When examining the left axilla in the sitting position, the patient may rest her (or his) left hand on your right shoulder while you explore the axilla with your right hand. Abduct the arm gently by supporting the patient's wrist with your right hand and examining with the other hand. Feel for the anterior group of nodes along the posterior border of the anterior axillary fold, the central group against the lateral chest wall and the posterior group along the posterior axillary fold. Finally, palpate along the medial border of the humerus to check for the lateral group of nodes. If you feel nodes, assess the size, shape, consistency, mobility and tenderness.

Abnormal palpation

BREAST LUMPS

A fibroadenoma is usually felt as a discrete, firm and smooth lump that is mobile in its surrounding tissue (endearingly referred to as a 'breast mouse'). Fibroadenosis is a bilateral condition characterised by 'lumpiness' of the breasts, which may be tender, especially in the premenstrual and menstrual phases of the cycle. Cancerous lesions usually feel hard and irregular and may be fixed to the skin or the underlying chest wall muscle.

BREAST ABSCESS (MASTITIS)

The temperature is raised and the skin of the infected breasts inflamed. If an abscess forms, you usually feel an extremely tender fluctuant mass.

ABNORMAL NIPPLE AND AREOLA

A bloodstained nipple discharge suggests an intraductal carcinoma or benign papilloma. Unilateral retraction or distortion of a nipple should also alert you to the possibility of malignancy. A unilateral red, crusty and scaling areola suggests Paget's disease of the breast.

PALPABLE LYMPH NODES

Suspect malignancy if the nodes are hard, nontender or fixed. Infection of axillary hair follicles or breast tissue may cause tender lymphadenitis.

SYMPTOMS OF GENITAL TRACT DISEASE

Menstrual history

ESTABLISH THE AGE OF THE MENARCHE

Most European and North American girls start menstruating by the age of 14.5 years (range 9–16 years). Menarche occurs at an average weight of 48 kg. By the age of 14 years, secondary sexual characteristics should have appeared. If the menarche has not occurred and there are no other signs of sexual development, it is reasonable to consider organic causes of primary amenorrhoea, such as gonadal dysgenesis (Turner's syndrome), congenital anatomical abnormalities of the genital tract (e.g. absence, uterine hypoplasia, vaginal hypoplasia), polycystic ovaries or pituitary or hypothalamic tumours in childhood. If secondary sexual characteristics have appeared, reassure the patient that investigation is usually only necessary if the menarche has not occurred by the age of 16 years.

DETERMINE THE PATTERN OF THE MENSTRUAL CYCLE

This cycle may vary from 21 to 35 days in normal women but the average duration is 28 days. Most healthy, fertile women have regular, predictable cycles that vary in duration by 1 or 2 days. Once regular periods are established, concern is soon aroused if there is deviation from the norm.

Cycles may be infrequent and scanty (oligomenorrhoea), unusually frequent (polymenorrhoea), excessively heavy (menorrhagia) or frequent and heavy (polymenorrhagia). Bleeding after intercourse is termed postcoital bleeding. If regular cycles are interrupted by days of spotting or blood-tinged discharge, this is known as intermenstrual bleeding.

Questions to ask
The menstrual cycle

- Age of menarche?
- Age of telarche?
- Do you use the contraceptive pill or hormone replacement therapy?
- Length of cycle?
- Days of blood loss?
- Number of tampons or pads used per day?
- Are there clots?
- Has there been a change in the periodicity of the cycle?

SECONDARY AMENORRHOEA

Differential diagnosis
Secondary amenorrhoea

Physiological
- Pregnancy
- Lactation

Psychological
- Anorexia nervosa
- Depression
- Fear of pregnancy

Hormonal
- Postcontraceptive pill
- Pituitary tumours
- Hyperthyroidism
- Adrenal tumours

Ovarian
- Polycystic ovaries
- Ovarian tumour
- Ovarian tuberculosis
- Constitutional disease
- Severe acute illness
- Chronic infections or illnesses
- Autoimmune diseases

ABNORMAL PATTERNS OF UTERINE BLEEDING

Oligomenorrhoea   The term used to describe infrequent or scanty menstrual periods.

Dysfunctional uterine bleeding   This term is used to describe frequent bleeding or excessive menstrual loss that cannot be ascribed to local pelvic pathology (e.g. fibroids, pelvic inflammatory disease, carcinoma, polyps).

Intermenstrual and postmenopausal bleeding   Patients may complain of vaginal bleeding unexpectedly between normal periods or after the menopause.

VAGINAL DISCHARGE

Many women notice slight soiling of the underwear at the end of the day; this is a normal physiological response to the cyclical changes occurring in the glandular epithelium of the genital tract and it is likely to become more profuse in pregnancy. A physiological discharge is scanty, mucoid and odourless. Pathological discharge is usually trichomonal or candidal vaginitis. The discharge may irritate the vulval skin, causing itching (pruritus vulvae) or burning.

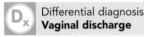

Dx Differential diagnosis
Vaginal discharge

Physiological
- Pregnancy
- Sexual arousal
- Menstrual cycle variation

Pathological
- Vaginal
  – candidosis (thrush)
  – trichomoniasis
  – Gardnerella associated
  – other bacteria (e.g. caused by a retained tampon)
  – postmenopausal vaginitis
- Cervical
  – gonorrhoea
  – nonspecific genital infection
  – herpes
  – cervical ectopy
  – cervical neoplasm (e.g. polyp)
  – intrauterine contraceptive device

PAIN

If the pain predictably occurs immediately before and during a period, the likely cause is dysmenorrhoea. Severe dysmenorrhoea should alert you to the possibility of endometriosis.

Ovulation may cause a unilateral iliac fossa or suprapubic pain in midcycle that lasts a few hours (mittelschmertz). Severe iliac fossa pain should warn you of the possibility of a haemorrhage into an ovarian cyst or torsion of a cyst. If the pain is preceded by a missed period, and if there is shock, you should also consider the possibility of a ruptured ectopic pregnancy. If the lower abdominal pain is accompanied by a vaginal discharge, fever, anorexia and nausea, consider acute infection of the fallopian tubes (acute salpingitis).

DYSPAREUNIA

Assess whether the pain is superficial (suggesting a local vulval cause or a psychological spasm) or deep (suggesting inflammatory or malignant disease of the cervix, uterus or adnexae). After the menopause, the vulva and vaginal become dry and atrophic and this may cause discomfort on intercourse.

Psychosexual history

Questions to ask
Psychosexual history

- Are you able to develop satisfying emotional relationships?
- Do you have satisfying physical relationships?
- Are you heterosexual, homosexual or ambivalent?
- Do you use contraception and, if so, what form?
- Do you have problems achieving arousal?
- Do you experience orgasm?

Obstetric history

Questions to ask
Obstetric history

- Have you ever been pregnant and, if so, how often?
- Did you have any problems falling pregnant?
- How many children do you have?
- Have you miscarried and, if so, at what stage of pregnancy?

Questions to ask
Obstetric history – *(cont'd)*

- Were there any complications in pregnancy (e.g. high blood pressure or diabetes)?
- Was the labour normal or did you require forceps assistance or a caesarean section?

EXAMINATION OF THE FEMALE GENITAL TRACT

Before the examination ask the patient to empty her bladder.

General examination

Before examining the genital tract you should perform a general examination. Excessive facial hair (hirsutism) may be normal but if overly excessive may provide a clue to an endocrine imbalance. Anaemia may occur with menstrual disorders and you may recognise syndromes that are commonly associated with menstrual disorders (e.g. thyrotoxicosis, myxoedema, Cushing's syndrome, anorexia nervosa, other serious chronic diseases).

Examination of the abdomen

Lower abdominal tenderness occurs in pelvic inflammatory disease and enlargement of the uterus or ovaries may present with a palpable lower abdominal mass. Large ovarian cysts may fill the abdomen; this presentation is readily mistaken for ascites (Fig. 8.3).

THE ABDOMEN IN PREGNANCY

After the 12th week of the pregnancy, the uterus becomes palpable above the symphysis pubis, making it possible to assess the maturity of the fetus from the height of the fundus (Fig. 8.4).

Examining the external genitalia

INSPECTION AND PALPATION OF THE VULVA

The pattern of hair distribution over the mons pubis provides a useful measure of sexual development. Once puberty is complete the mons and outer aspects of the labia majora should be well covered with hair. Systematically examine the labia majora, labia minora, the introitus, urethra and clitoris.

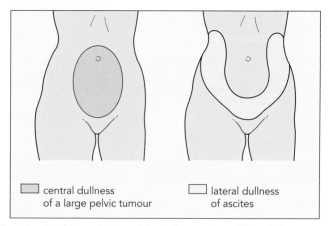

| | central dullness of a large pelvic tumour | | lateral dullness of ascites |

Fig. 8.3 Careful examination of the abdomen allows differentiation between large ovarian cysts and ascites. An ovarian cyst displaces the bowel towards the flanks: the central abdomen is dull, whereas the flanks are more resonant. This contrasts with ascites, in which the flanks are dull and the central abdomen tympanitic.

week	height of uterus
12	palpable above pubic bone
16	midway between symphysis and umbilicus
20	lower border of umbilicus
28	midway between umbilicus and xiphisternum
34	just below xiphisternum
38–40	height drops as fetal head engages pelvis

Fig. 8.4 The maturity of a pregnancy can be assessed by examining the height of the fundus.

Gently separate the labia with the fingers of your left hand and inspect the medial aspect. Palpate the length of the labia majora between index finger and thumb. A normal Bartholin's gland is not palpable.

To expose the vestibule, separate the labia minora, which exposes the vaginal orifice and urethra.

After the menopause the skin and subcutaneous tissue of the external genitalia become atrophic and the mucosa loses its moist texture.

ABNORMALITIES OF THE VULVA

A confluent, itchy, red rash on the inner aspects of the thighs and extending to the labia suggests candidiasis. This is often associated with a vaginal discharge.

The vulva is a common site for boils (furuncles) to appear. These are tender to palpation.

Crops of small, painful, vulval and perianal papules and vesicles that ulcerate suggest a herpes simplex infection. You may notice multiple genital warts (condylomata acuminata), which can coalesce to form large irregular tissue masses. The lesions usually occur on the fourchette and may extend onto the labia, and posteriorly onto the perineum. Flat, round or oval papules covered by a grey exudate suggest lesions of secondary syphilis (condylomata lata).

The most common ulcerating lesions include carcinoma of the vulva or macerated, ulcerating herpetic warts.

Leucoplakia is a potentially malignant, hypertrophic skin lesion affecting the labia, clitoris and perineum. The skin thickens, feels hard and indurated and is distinguished from surrounding tissue by its white colour.

Differential diagnosis
Vulval ulceration

Squamous cell carcinoma
Infections
- Syphilitic chancre
- Secondary syphilis
- Granuloma inguinale (chlamydia)
- Chancroid (*Haemophilus ducreyi*)
- Ulcerating herpetic warts

Behçet's syndrome

Examination of the vagina

Separate the labia to expose the vestibule and ask the patient to 'bear down' and exert a downward force on the vulva. If there is muscle weakness, the posterior bladder wall may prolapse, causing a bulge (a cystocele) along the anterior vaginal wall. If the rectum prolapses, this may cause a bulge (a rectocele) in the posterior vaginal wall. Uterine prolapse may also occur.

A full vaginal examination includes inspection with a speculum, followed by a bimanual examination of the uterus and adnexae.

SPECULUM EXAMINATION

A bivalve speculum (e.g. Cusco's) is the instrument most commonly used to inspect the vagina.

Adjust the light source to illuminate the vagina. Make any minor adjustments necessary to establish the optimal position for visualising the cervix.

Examination of the cervix

The position of the cervix relates to the position of the uterus (Fig. 8.5). The shape of the external os changes after childbirth. In nulliparous women, the os is round, whereas after childbirth, the os may be slit-like or stellate.

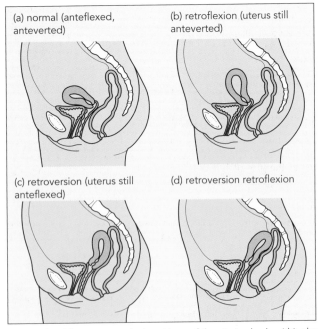

(a) normal (anteflexed, anteverted)

(b) retroflexion (uterus still anteverted)

(c) retroversion (uterus still anteflexed)

(d) retroversion retroflexion

Fig. 8.5 The different anatomical positions of the uterine body within the pelvis. (a) The normal uterus is angled forward from the plane of the vagina (anteverted) and bends forward on itself (anteflexed). In some women the uterus assumes different positions: (b) retroflexed, anteverted; (c) retroverted, anteflexed; (d) retroverted, retroflexed.

The surface of the cervix is pink, smooth and regular, and resembles the epithelium of the vagina. In early pregnancy the cervix has a bluish colour caused by increased vascularity (Chadwick's sign). During pregnancy, the squamocolumnar junction may migrate beyond the external os and onto the cervix, retreating back, a few months after childbirth, into the cervical canal. Periodically, after pregnancy, the squamocolumnar junctions fail to regress into the os, giving the appearance of an erosion (ectopy). Cervical 'erosions' are not ulcerated surfaces but a term used to describe the appearance of the cervix when the endocervical epithelium extends onto the outer surface of the cervix. The columnar epithelium appears as a strawberry-red area spreading circumferentially around the os or onto the anterior or posterior lips. Cervical ectopy cannot be confidently distinguished from early cervical cancer, so cytology should always be performed.

ABNORMALITIES OF THE CERVIX

Nabothian cysts may develop. These are small, round, raised white or yellow lesions which only assume importance if they become infected. There may be a cervical discharge. If there is a pungent odour, suspect an infective cause and swab the area. An inflamed cervix covered by a mucopurulent discharge or slough is characteristic of acute and chronic cervicitis. Cherry-red friable polyps may grow from the cervix (a source of vaginal bleeding after intercourse). Ulceration and fungating growths suggest cervical carcinoma.

Internal examination of the uterus

The speculum examination is followed by the vaginal examination. Expose the introitus by separating the labia with the thumb and fore-finger of the gloved left hand and gently introduce the gloved and lubricated right index and middle fingers into the vagina (Fig. 8.6).

CERVIX

It should feel firm, rounded and smooth. Assess the mobility of the cervix by moving it gently and palpate the fornices.

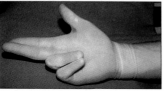

Fig. 8.6 The finger position used for performing a vaginal examination.

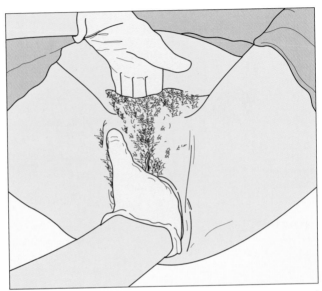

Fig. 8.7 The bimanual technique used to palpate the uterus. The vaginal fingers lift the cervix, while the other hand dips downwards and inwards to meet the fundus.

Abnormalities of the cervix

In pregnancy, the cervix softens (Hegar's sign). If there is tenderness on movement (known as 'excitation tenderness'), suspect infection or inflammation of the uterus or adnexae; or if the patient is shocked, suspect an ectopic pregnancy.

UTERUS

A bimanual technique is used to assess the size and position of the organ (Fig. 8.7). An anteverted fundus should be palpable just above the symphysis. Assess its size, consistency and mobility, and note any masses and tenderness.

Abnormalities of the uterus

If the uterus appears to be uniformly enlarged, consider a pregnancy, fibroid or endometrial tumour. Single, large uterine fibroids are felt on abdominal examination as a firm, nontender, well-defined rounded mass arising from the pelvis. On bimanual palpation, the mass appears contiguous with the cervix: the two structures move together.

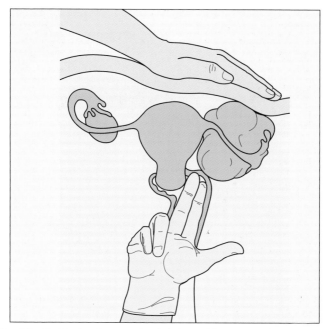

Fig. 8.8 Positioning the vaginal and abdominal fingers to palpate the adnexal structures.

ADNEXAE

Gently but firmly appose the fingers of either hand by pressing the abdominal hand inward and downward, and the vaginal fingers upwards and laterally. Feel for the adnexal structures as the interposed tissues slip between your fingers (Fig. 8.8). If you feel an adnexal structure, assess its size, shape, mobility and tenderness. Ovaries are firm, ovoid, and often palpable. Normal fallopian tubes are impalpable.

Abnormalities of the adnexal structures

The most common causes of enlarged ovaries include benign cysts (e.g. follicular or corpus luteal cysts) and malignant ovarian tumours. Ovarian tumours are either unilateral or bilateral. Cysts feel smooth and the wall may be compressible. Occasionally, ovarian tumours are large enough to be palpable on abdominal examination and may fill the lower and mid-abdomen, creating the impression of ascites.

In acute infections of the fallopian tubes (salpingitis), there is lower abdominal tenderness and guarding, and, on vaginal examination, marked tenderness of the lateral fornices and cervix. In chronic salpingitis, the lower abdomen and lateral fornices are tender, yet the uterus and adnexae may be amenable to examination. If the tubes are blocked, there may be cystic swelling of the tubes (hydrosalpinx) or they may become infected and purulent (pyosalpinx).

After completing the bimanual examination, withdraw your fingers from the vagina and inspect the glove tips for blood or discharge.

 Examination of elderly people
Breasts and genital tract

- There is rapid fall in sex hormone synthesis after the menopause, resulting in changes in the structure and function of the genitalia
- There is progressive involution of the breast tissue and, as the acinar tissue atrophies, the breasts become more pendulous
- The risk of breast cancer remains at any age, including the very old
- After the menopause there is loss of vulval adipose tissue, and reduction in vaginal secretion results in drying of the mucosal surface
- The atrophy of tissue of the introitus results in vestibular narrowing, increased susceptibility to urinary tract infection and dyspareunia
- Loss of sex hormones results in altered hair distribution and androgen dominance may be apparent, with male pattern facial hair growth, mild to moderate male pattern baldness and loss of the female pattern labial hairline
- Despite involutional changes, many older women maintain libido and remain sexually active into the later years of life
- Atrophy of the vagina and introitus can be prevented by hormone replacement therapy and topical oestrogen application
- Vaginal lubrication can be enhanced by using water-soluble lubricant jellies

Review
The gynaecological examination

General examination
- Endocrine syndrome
- Hirsutism, acne
- Breast examination
- Routine abdominal examination
- Inguinal lymph nodes

Vulva
- Inspection and palpation of the vulva
- Bartholin's gland palpation

Vagina
- Digital examination
  - cervix
  - cervical tenderness
  - fornices
  - pouch of Douglas

Uterus
- Bimanual palpation
  - body and fundus
  - adnexal region
  - ovaries

Speculum
- Inspect cervix and os
- Take cervical smear
- Bacterial swab for culture
- Inspect vaginal mucosa as speculum withdrawn

9.
The Male Genitalia

SYMPTOMS OF GENITAL TRACT DISEASE

Urethral Discharge

A discharge of smegma from a normal prepuce is very different from a discharge caused by urethritis. In urethritis, the patient may complain of urinary symptoms such as burning or stinging when passing urine. Ask about a recent episode of gastroenteritis, for urethritis may follow a few weeks later. Reiter's syndrome is the most florid manifestation of this association and is characterised by a urethral discharge, balanitis, painful joints (arthritis and tendinitis) and bilateral conjunctivitis.

Questions to ask
Urethral discharge

- Is there a possibility of recent exposure to a sexually transmitted disease?
- How long ago might you have had such a contact (incubation period)?
- Does your partner complain of a vaginal discharge?
- Have you experienced joint pains or gritty, red eyes?
- Have you recently suffered from gastroenteritis?

Differential diagnosis
Urethral discharge

Physiological
- Sexual arousal

Pathological
- Gonococcal urethritis (incubation 2–6 days)
- Nongonococcal urethritis
- Idiopathic nonspecific urethritis

- *Chlamydia trachomatis*
- *Trichomonas vaginalis*
- *Candida albicans*
- Posturinary catheter
- Reiter's syndrom (may follow gastroenteritis) includes arthritis and conjunctivitis

Genital ulcers

Enquire about possible contact with sexually transmitted disease or casual sexual encounters. Ask whether the ulcer is painful and try to assess a possible incubation period. Herpetic ulcers tend to recur and may be preceded by a prodrome of a prickly sensation or pain in the loins. Sexual transmission may affect the mouth or anus as well as the penis. Exotic ulcerating venereal infections occur in the tropics and it is important to obtain a history of foreign travel and possible sexual contact.

Testicular pain

Inflammation or trauma to the testes causes an intense visceral pain that may radiate towards the groin and abdomen. The pain may be accompanied by swelling and be aggravated by movement or even light palpation. Painless swelling of a testis should alert you to the possibility of a cystic lesion or malignancy.

Differential diagnosis
Testicular pain

- Trauma
- Infection (mumps orchitis)
- Epididymitis
- Testicular torsion
- Torsion of epididymal cyst

Impotence

The term refers to a spectrum of sexual dysfunction ranging from loss of libido, failure to obtain or to maintain an erection, to inability to achieve orgasm. Impotence is often a manifestation of emotional disturbance. Take a careful drug and alcohol history; alcoholism is an important cause of impotence and many widely prescribed drugs are associated with impotence. An obvious association with organic disease may be apparent in patients presenting with concomitant cardiovascular, respiratory or neurological symptoms.

Infertility

Primary infertility refers to a failure to achieve conception, whereas secondary infertility refers to a difficulty or a failure to conceive,

Questions to ask
Infertility

- Have you or your partner ever conceived?
- Do you have difficulty obtaining or maintaining an erection?
- Do you ejaculate?
- Do you understand the timing of ovulation in your partner?
- Are you on any medication that may cause impotence or sperm malfunction (e.g. sulfasalazine)?
- Have you noticed any change in facial hair growth?
- Have you ever had cancer treatment?

although there has been at least one successful conception in the past. Male infertility accounts for approximately one-third of childless relationships.

EXAMINATION OF THE MALE GENITALIA

The genitalia are usually examined with the patient lying but remember that varicoceles and scrotal hernias may only be apparent when the patient stands.

GENERAL EXAMINATION

In testicular malfunction (hypogonadism), there may be loss of axillary hair, the pubic hair distribution may start to resemble the

Differential diagnosis
Male gynaecomastia

Physiological
- Puberty
- Old age

Pathological
- Hypogonadism
- Liver cirrhosis
- Drugs (spironolactone, digoxin, oestrogens)
- Tumours (bronchogenic carcinoma, adrenal carcinoma, testicular tumours)
- Thyrotoxicosis

distinctive female pattern and there is a typical facial appearance with wrinkling around the mouth. You will have also checked the breast and noted whether or not gynaecomastia was evident.

Normal penis

Gently retract the foreskin (prepuce) to expose the glans penis. The foreskin should be supple, allowing smooth and painless retraction. There is often a trace of odourless, curd-like smegma underlying the foreskin. Examine the external urethral meatus. If the patient has complained of a urethral discharge, try to elicit this sign. If a discharge appears, swab the area with a sterile bud.

Abnormalities of the penis

Prepuce   The prepuce may be too tight to retract over the glans (phimosis). If the prepuce is tight but retracts and catches behind the glans, oedema and swelling may occur, preventing the return of the foreskin (paraphimosis).

Glans   Hypospadias is a developmental abnormality causing the urethral meatus to appear on the inferior (ventral) surface of the glans (primary hypospadias), penis (secondary hypospadias) or even the perineum (tertiary hypospadias). Inflammation of the glans is termed balanitis; if there is inflammation of the glans and prepuce, the term balanoposthitis is used. Genital (herpetic) warts may be seen on the glans.

Urethral discharge   The cause of a urethral discharge cannot be confidently predicted from appearance, although gonorrhoea is likely to cause a profuse purulent discharge. Nongonococcal urethritis may also be caused by urethral infection or be associated with Reiter's syndrome.

Penile ulcers   Examine the ulcer and always palpate the groins for inguinal lymph node involvement because the skin of the penis drains to this group of nodes. The most common cause is herpetic ulceration. Characteristic painless vesicles occur 4–5 days after sexual contact. The vesicles often rupture, causing painful superficial erosions with a characteristic erythematous halo. The confluence of these erosions may cause discrete ulcers that can become secondarily infected. Consider syphilis (primary chancre) (Fig. 9.1) and in the tropics consider chancroid, lymphogranuloma venereum and granuloma inguinale. Infrequently, fixed drug reactions may cause penile ulceration. Squamous cell carcinoma may present as an ulcer of the penis or the scrotum.

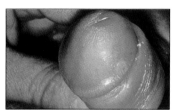

Fig. 9.1 The primary chancre of syphilis may occur on the glans, prepuce or shaft.

 Differential diagnosis
Genital ulcers

Infections
- Genital herpes
- Syphilis (chancre, mucous patches, gumma)
- Tropical ulcers

Balanitis
- Severe candidiasis
- Circinate balanitis (Reiter's syndrome)

Drug eruption
- Localised fixed drug eruption
- Generalised (Stevens–Johnson syndrome)

Carcinoma
Behçet's syndrome

Priapism Painful and prolonged erection is termed priapism. Most often there is no obvious cause but predisposing factors such as leukaemia, haemoglobinopathies (e.g. sickle cell anaemia) and drugs (aphrodisiacs) should be considered.

Examination of the scrotum

The left testis lies lower than the right. Feel the testicle between your thumb and first two fingers (Fig. 9.2). Note the size and consistency of the testis. Next, palpate the epididymis, which is felt as an elongated structure along the posterolateral surface of the testicle (Fig. 9.3). The epididymis is broadest superiorly at its head. Finally, roll with the finger and thumb the vas deferens, which passes from the tail of the epididymis to the inguinal canal through the external inguinal canal.

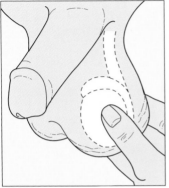

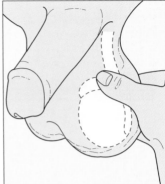

Fig. 9.2 Palpate the testis between your thumb and first two fingers.

Fig. 9.3 The epididymis is felt along the posterior pole of the testis.

ABNORMALITIES OF THE SCROTUM

If one-half of the scrotum appears smooth and poorly developed, consider an undescended testis (cryptorchidism). This appearance of the scrotum helps to distinguish a maldescent from a retractile testis, in which the testis has descended but retracts vigorously towards the external inguinal ring.

The scrotal skin may be red and inflamed; a common cause is candidiasis. Small yellowish scrotal lumps or nodules are common and usually represent sebaceous cysts.

Swellings in the scrotum

Decide whether the swelling arises from an indirect inguinal hernia or from the scrotal contents. It is possible to 'get above' a testicular swelling but not a scrotal hernia (Fig. 9.4). An intrinsic swelling may arise from enlargement of the testis, testicular appendages and epididymis or by an accumulation of fluid in the tunica vaginalis.

Cystic swelling   Cystic accumulations are caused by entrapment of fluid in the tunica vaginalis (a hydrocele) or accumulation of fluid in an epididymal cyst and are typically fluctant. The tense fluid-filled cyst will fluctuate between finger and thumb in response to the pressure change. Cystic lesions usually transilluminate. Next, try to distinguish between a hydrocele and an epididymal cyst. As the epididymis lies behind the body of the testis, an epididymal cyst is felt

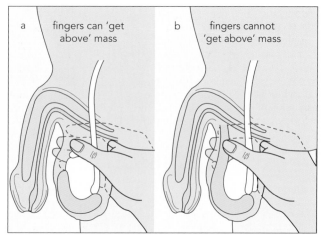

Fig. 9.4 It is possible to 'get above' a true scrotal swelling (a), whereas this is not possible if the swelling is caused by an inguinal hernia that has descended into the scrotum (b).

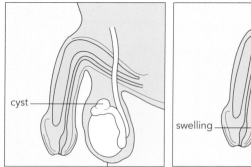

Fig. 9.5 An epididymal cyst is felt separately from the testis and lies posteriorly.

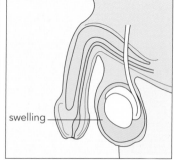

Fig. 9.6 A hydrocele surrounds the entire testis, which cannot, therefore, be felt as a discrete organ.

as a distinct swelling behind the adjoining testis (Fig. 9.5). In contrast, a hydrocele surrounds and envelops the testis, which becomes impalpable as a discrete organ (Fig. 9.6).

Varicocele Varicoceles are almost always left–sided. A varicocele results from a varicosity of the veins of the pampiniform plexus. Most varicoceles do not cause symptoms and are discovered as an incidental finding. However, a patient may rarely present with scrotal swelling, discomfort or infertility. Examine the patient in the standing position; the varicocele feels like a 'bag of worms'. Ask the patient to cough while you palpate the varicocele; a characteristic feature is transmission of the raised intra-abdominal pressure to the varicocele, which is felt as a discrete cough impulse. The varicocele is separate from the testis. A varicocele usually empties when the patient lies supine.

Solid swellings Diffuse, acutely painful swelling usually occurs in acute inflammatory condition such as orchitis or torsion of the testis. Solid masses may be smooth or craggy, tender or painless but, whatever the character, carcinoma must be the first differential diagnosis. Other solid masses include tuberculomas and syphilitic gummas. Solid tumours of the epididymis are due to chronic inflammation (usually tuberculous epididymitis) and are generally benign.

Torsion of the testis
This usually occurs in young boys and presents with severe scrotal pain that generally radiates to the inguinal region and lower abdomen. On examination, the scrotal skin overlying the affected testis may be reddened, with the affected testis lying higher than the unaffected testis. The testis may be very tender and the spermatic cord may feel thickened and sensitive to palpation.

Examination of the lymphatics

The skin lymphatics of the penis and scrotum drain towards the inguinal nodes; complete your genital examination by feeling for nodes in the groin, which are felt deep to the inguinal crease. The testicular lymphatics drain to intra-abdominal nodes. Special tests such as computerised tomography or lymphangiography are necessary to evaluate the testicular lymphatics.

ENLARGED INGUINAL NODES
Enlarged nodes occur in infective and malignant disorders affecting the skin of the penis and scrotum. The primary chancre of syphilis is usually associated with lymphadenopathy. The most florid forms of inguinal lymphadenopathy occur in patients with lymphogranuloma venereum.

Examination of elderly people
Genitalia in elderly males

- Men remain sexually active well into the later years of life
- Impotence and loss of libido commonly accompany chronic disease such as heart failure and respiratory and renal/prostatic disease
- Always consider drugs when elderly patients complain of impotence or loss of libido (e.g. antihypertensive medication)
- While women stop ovulating by the sixth decade, most men continue to produce sperm well into the eighth and ninth decades
- Benign prostatic hypertrophy of its own accord does not affect genital function; prostatectomy may result in retrograde ejaculation or nerve damage and impotence
- Hydrocele and varicocele are common causes of testicular swelling in elderly men but testicular cancer is rare

Review
Examination of the male genitalia

- Note pattern of hair distribution
- Stage sexual development
- Examine abdomen generally
- Examine inguinal lymph nodes
- Inguinal hernias?
- Retract foreskin
- Examine glans penis and meatus
- Check for urethral discharge
- Examine the scrotum
  - inspect scrotal skin
  - check lie of testes (left lower than right)
  - palpate the testes and epididymis
  - check scrotal swellings for fluctuation and transillumination
  - palpate the spermatic cord within the scrotum

10.
Bone, Joint and Muscle

SYMPTOMS OF BONE, JOINT AND MUSCLE DISORDERS

Bone

PAIN
- Deep, boring quality
- May be focal (tumour, infection, fracture)
- May be diffuse (osteoporosis, osteomalacia).

Joint

PAIN
- Usually the most prominent complaint of arthritic disorders.
- Referred to segments (sclerotomes) which differ from dermatomes (Fig. 10.1).
- Hence joint pain can be felt at some distance from the affected structure.
- Osteoarthritis and rheumatoid arthritis typically result in chronic pain with periodic exacerbations.
- Septic arthritis or gout produce an acutely painful joint.
- Inflammatory joint disease tends to cause pain on waking, improving with activity but returning at rest.

Differential diagnosis
Bone pain

Focal
- Fracture or trauma
- Infection
- Malignancy
- Paget's disease
- Osteoid osteoma

Diffuse
- Malignancy
- Paget's disease
- Osteomalacia
- Osteoporosis
- Metabolic bone disease

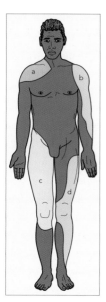

Fig. 10.1 Distribution of pain arising from (a) the acromioclavicular or sternoclavicular joints, (b) the scapulohumeral joint, (c) the hip joint and (d) the knee joint.

- Mechanical joint disease (e.g. due to osteoarthritis) leads to pain that worsens during the course of the day, particularly with activity.

SWELLING AND CREPITUS
- Elicit the duration of any swelling, whether it is painful and whether it fluctuates.
- Crepitus is a grating noise or sensation.
- Fine crepitus is more readily felt than heard.
- Readily audible crepitus is associated with advanced degeneration in large joints.

Dx Differential diagnosis
Causes of joint pain

- Inflammatory
  - rheumatoid arthritis
  - ankylosing spondylitis
- Mechanical
  - osteoarthritis
- Infective
  - pyogenic
  - tuberculosis
  - brucellosis
- Traumatic

LOCKING
- Occurs when ectopic material becomes interposed between the articular surfaces.
- Particularly prevalent with knee cartilage damage.

Muscle

Muscle symptoms include pain, stiffness, spontaneous movements and cramps.

 Differential diagnosis
Causes of muscle pain

- Inflammatory
  – polymyositis
  – dermatomyositis
- Infective
  – pyogenic
  – cysticercosis
- Traumatic
- Polymyalgia rheumatica
- Neuropathic, e.g.
  Guillain–Barré syndrome

PAIN AND STIFFNESS
- Muscle pain tends to be deep, constant and poorly localised.
- Muscle stiffness is usually the consequence of unaccustomed activity. If it persists, suspect spasticity.

WEAKNESS

WASTING AND FASCICULATION
- Determine the duration of these symptoms and their distribution.

CRAMPS
- Usually physiological but can occur in metabolic myopathies.

GENERAL PRINCIPLES OF EXAMINATION

Bone

- Expose structure.
- Assess deformity and tenderness.
- Assess any altered temperature.

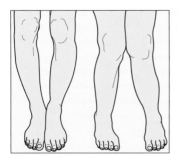

Fig. 10.2 Genu varum (left) and genu valgum (right).

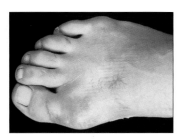

Fig. 10.3 Acute gout of the first metatarsophalangeal joint.

Joint

INSPECTION
Swelling
- Determine if within or adjacent to the joint.
- Causes include effusions, synovial thickening (e.g. rheumatoid arthritis) and bony deformity.

Deformity
- Results either from misalignment of the bones forming the joint or from alteration of the relationship between the articular surfaces.
- Valgus deformity – deviation of part distal to the joint away from the midline (Fig. 10.2).
- Varus deformity – deviation of part distal to the joint towards the midline (Fig. 10.2).
- Subluxation – partial loss of contact of the articulatory surfaces.
- Dislocation – complete loss of contact of the articulatory surfaces.

Skin changes
Redness of the skin over a joint implies an underlying acute inflammatory process (e.g. gout or septic arthritis) (Fig. 10.3).

Changes of adjacent structure

The most striking change adjacent to a diseased joint is muscle wasting.

PALPATION

During palpation of a joint, assess the nature of any swelling, whether there is tenderness, and whether the joint is hot.

Swelling

Is the swelling:

- Hard? – suggesting bone deformities secondary to osteoarthritis.
- Spongy? – suggesting synovial thickening, e.g. rheumatoid arthritis.
- Fluctuant? – an effusion can be displaced from one part of the joint to another.

Tenderness

Determine whether any tenderness is focal or diffuse. In an acutely inflamed joint, the whole of the contour is tender. If there is derangement of a single knee cartilage, tenderness is confined to the cartilage margin.

Temperature

- For a small joint, assess temperature with the finger tips.
- For a larger joint, e.g. the knee, rub the back of your hand across the joint then compare it with its fellow.

MOVEMENT

- To define the range of joint movement, start with the joint in the neutral position:
  - the lower limbs extended with the feet dorsiflexed to 90°
  - the upper limbs midway between pronation and supination with the arms flexed to 90° at the elbows.
- Active joint movement is that initiated by the patient.
- Passive joint movement is that induced by the examiner.
- From the neutral position, record the degrees of flexion and extension.
- If extension does not normally occur at a joint (e.g. the knee) but is present, describe the movement as hyperextension and give its range in degrees.
- Restricted movement, say of knee extension, is recorded as X° flexion deformity or as X° lack of extension.
- For a ball-and-socket joint, record flexion, extension, abduction, and internal and external rotation.

Muscle

Initial assessment will include inspection, palpation then testing of muscle power.

INSPECTION

Look for evidence of muscle wasting, signs of abnormal muscle bulk and for spontaneous contractions.

Wasting

If not due to adjacent joint disease, or a global loss of body weight, reflects either primary muscle disease or disease of its innervating neuron.

Increased muscle bulk

Rare.

- True hypertrophy – seen in some forms of congenital myotonia.
- Pseudohypertrophy – due to fatty infiltration. The muscle is actually weak. Seen in some forms of muscular dystrophy (e.g. Duchenne's).

Spontaneous muscle contractions

Seen in both upper and lower motor neuron disorders.

- Flexor or extensor spasms – typically affecting the hips, knees or both. Seen with spinal disorders, e.g. multiple sclerosis.
- Fasciculation – episodic twitching due to contraction of muscle fibres supplied by a single motor unit. It is seen with motor neuron disease but can also occur in normal individuals.

PALPATION

Muscle palpation is of limited value. Look for tenderness. It is seen in muscle infection, inflammatory muscle disease (e.g. polymyositis) and in certain neuropathies (e.g. due to beriberi).

MUSCLE POWER

Use the MRC classification of muscle power.

- Is the weakness global or focal?
- If focal, can it be explained by a root or peripheral nerve lesion?
- Is the weakness fluctuant?

Symptoms and signs
MRC classification of muscle power

5 Normal
4 Contracts against resistance but incomplete
3 Contracts against gravity but not resistance
2 Contracts with gravity eliminated
1 Flicker of contraction
0 Nil

REGIONAL EXAMINATION

Temporomandibular joints

- Assess the range of movement and whether there is local tenderness.
- The joints lie immediately in front of and below the tragus.

Spine

- Ask the patient to undress to his or her underwear.
- Inspect the whole spine.
- Palpate the spine for tenderness.
- Assess the range of movement.

CERVICAL SPINE
- Examine the patient sitting.
- Test flexion, extension, lateral flexion and rotation.
- Determine whether any movement causes pain, and whether that pain is referred to the arm or head.

THORACIC SPINE
- For movement, measure chest expansion.
- Then, with the patient's arms folded across the chest, ask the patient, while sitting, to twist as far as possible to one side then the other.

Symptoms and signs
Spinal deformities (Fig. 10.4)

Kyphosis – increased flexion
Lordosis – increase extension

Scoliosis – increased lateral curvature
Gibbus – focal flexion deformity

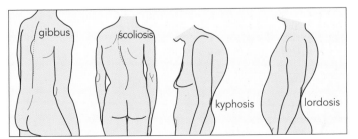

Fig. 10.4 Spinal deformities.

LUMBAR SPINE
- Ask the patient to touch the toes.
- Then test extension and lateral flexion.

SACROILIAC JOINTS
- Palpate the joints (they lie under the dimples found in the lower lumbar region).
- To test whether movement is painful, first press firmly over the midline of the sacrum with the patient prone, then, with the patient supine, forcibly flex one hip while maintaining the other hip extended.

Differential diagnosis
Back pain

- Muscle or ligamentous strain
- Degenerative disc disease
- Spondylolisthesis
- Arthritis – osteoarthritis, rheumatoid arthritis, ankylosing spondylitis
- Bone infection – pyogenic, tuberculous
- Trauma
- Osteochondritis
- Metabolic bone disease

NERVE STRETCH TESTS
Carried out to determine whether there is evidence of nerve root irritation, usually due to lumbar disc prolapse.

Straight leg raising (Fig. 10.5)
- Place the patient in the supine position. Lift each leg in turn at the hip. Normally 80° – 90° of hip flexion is possible.
- The test is positive with nerve root irritation at L4 or below.
- If the foot is returned to the neutral position, and the knee flexed, the hip can be flexed further without pain, but the pain reappears when the knee is then extended (Lasègue's test).

Femoral stretch (Fig. 10.6)
- Place patient in prone position. Flex the knee, then extend the leg at the hip.
- The test is positive with nerve root irritation at L2, 3 or 4.

CLINICAL APPLICATION
Prolapsed intervertebral disc
Most commonly in cervical (mainly 5/6 or 6/7) or lumbar (mainly 4/5 or 5/S1) region (Fig. 10.7).

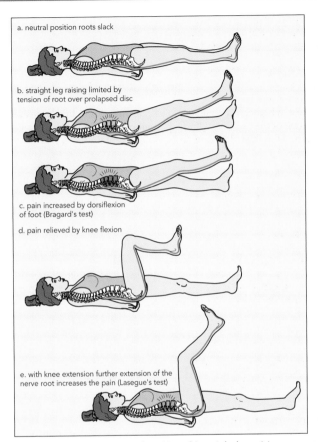

a. neutral position roots slack

b. straight leg raising limited by tension of root over prolapsed disc

c. pain increased by dorsiflexion of foot (Bragard's test)

d. pain relieved by knee flexion

e. with knee extension further extension of the nerve root increases the pain (Lasegue's test)

Fig. 10.5 Stretch tests: (a) neutral position, (b) straight leg raising, (c) Bragard's test, (d) knee flexion and (e) Lasegue's test.

Ankylosing spondylitis
The patient, usually male, complains of spinal pain and stiffness, the latter improving with exercise.

Rheumatoid arthritis
Frequently affects the upper cervical spine.

Spinal tumours
Usually metastatic from prostate, breast, bronchus or kidney.

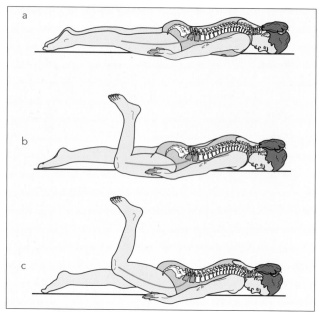

Fig. 10.6 (a) Femoral stretch. The pain may be triggered by (b) knee flexion alone or (c) in combination with hip extension.

Tuberculosis
Typically affects thoracolumbar region.

Trauma
- Cervical injuries include atlantoaxial dislocation, fractures of the arch of the atlas and compression fractures of the vertebral bodies.
- Thoracic and lumbar injuries include compression fractures and fractures of the transverse process. Pathological fractures commonly occur at these levels.

The shoulder

INSPECTION AND PALPATION
- Inspect the contour of the shoulder.
- Anterior dislocation results in forward and downward displacement with alteration of the shoulder contour.
- Posterior dislocation is obvious.

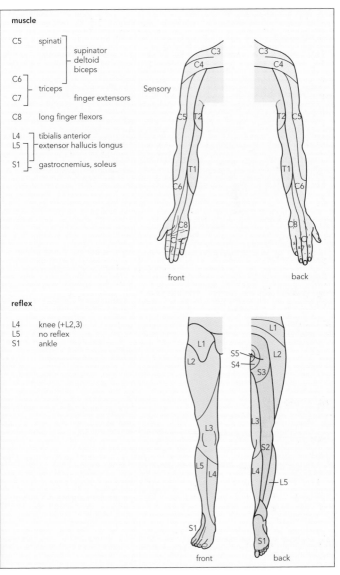

muscle

C5 spinati
                ⎤
      supinator │
    - deltoid   ⎥
      biceps   ⎦
C6 ⎤
   ⎢- triceps
C7 ⎦
      finger extensors
C8 long finger flexors

L4 ⎤ tibialis anterior
L5 ⎤⎦ extensor hallucis longus
S1 ⎦ gastrocnemius, soleus

Sensory

reflex

L4   knee (+L2,3)
L5   no reflex
S1   ankle

Fig. 10.7 Sensory, motor and reflex changes in cervical and lumbar root syndromes.

JOINT MOVEMENT
- Most movement involves both the glenohumeral joint and rotation of the scapula across the thorax.
- Test flexion, extension, internal and external rotation, abduction and adduction.

Clinical application
- Frozen shoulder – all movements are restricted.
- Painful arc syndrome – pain occurs during an arc of abduction of the shoulder, secondary to inflammation of one of the muscles of the rotator cuff or the subacromial bursa.
- Bicipital tendonitis – due to tenosynovitis of the long head of biceps. Causes pain in the anterior aspect of the shoulder and arm.
- Trauma – includes dislocation, fracture dislocation and fractures of the neck of the humerus.

MUSCLE FUNCTION
Test the power of supraspinatus, infraspinatus, deltoid, latissimus dorsi and pectoralis major.

Clinical application
- Cervical radiculopathy – affecting C5 will cause weakness of spinati, deltoid and biceps with depression of the biceps and supinator reflexes.
- Neuralgic amyotrophy – severe shoulder pain is followed by patchy weakness and wasting of the shoulder girdle muscles.
- Circumflex nerve palsy – results in deltoid weakness and a small area of sensory loss over the lateral aspect of the shoulder. Rare.

The elbow

INSPECTION AND PALPATION
- Inspect the joint from behind.
- Palpate the subcutaneous border of the ulna, then the medial and lateral epicondyles.

Clinical application
- Tennis elbow – inflammation of the origins of the forearm extensor muscles just below the lateral epicondyle.
- Golfer's elbow – inflammation of the origins of the forearm flexor muscles just below the medial epicondyle.
- Rheumatoid arthritis – rheumatoid nodules are commonly found along the subcutaneous border of the ulna.
- Trauma – includes dislocations and fractures of the radial head and distal humerus. Dislocation is usually in a posterolateral direction.

JOINT MOVEMENT

Test flexion, extension, supination and pronation.

MUSCLE FUNCTION

Test the power of the biceps, the triceps, the pronators and the supinators.

Clinical application

Cervical radiculopathy – affecting C6 will involve biceps, brachioradialis, supinator and part of triceps. The triceps reflex is the one usually most affected. Any sensory loss affects the thumb and index finger.

The forearm and wrist

INSPECTION AND PALPATION

- Compare the sizes of the forearms and wrists (the dominant forearm is generally rather wider).
- Look for any deformity and palpate for areas of tenderness.

JOINT MOVEMENT

Test wrist extension and flexion, then radial and ulnar deviation.

Clinical application

- Rheumatoid arthritis – wrist involvement is common in rheumatoid arthritis. Besides limitation of movement, stretching of the ulnar collateral ligament allows the head of the ulna to subluxate upwards (Fig. 10.8).
- Trauma – fractures usually occur through the distal radius or ulna, typically after a fall on an outstretched hand. Colles' fracture is sited about 1–2 cm above the distal end of the radius. The fracture is displaced dorsally. Smith's fracture, at the same site, produces displacement in the opposite direction.
- Osteoarthritis – commonly affects the carpometacarpal joint of the thumb.

MUSCLE FUNCTION

Test flexion and extension of the wrist, then the long finger flexors and extensors.

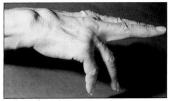

Fig. 10.8 Elevation of the ulnar head in rheumatoid arthritis. The flexion deformity of the fourth and fifth digits is the result of rupture of their extensor tendons.

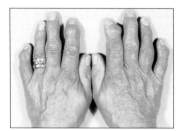

Fig. 10.9 The square hand of osteoarthritis.

Clinical application
- Cervical radiculopathy – C7 radiculopathy produces weakness of triceps, the wrist and finger extensors and depression of the triceps reflex. Any sensory loss is over the middle finger.
- Radial palsy – usually results from trauma to the nerve in the spiral groove. Affected muscles include supinator, brachioradialis, and the wrist and finger extensors. The brachioradialis component of the supinator reflex is depressed. Sensory loss, often slight, is confined to the region of the anatomical snuff box.

The hand

INSPECTION AND PALPATION
- A good way to examine the hands both for joint and muscle function is to ask the patient to sit opposite you with the hands spread out on a flat surface.
- Palpate the joints for tenderness and assess any swelling.
- Also inspect the skin, the nails and the tendons.

Clinical application
- Rheumatoid arthritis – principally affects the metacarpophalangeal and proximal interphalangeal joints. Later, deformity is accompanied by muscle wasting.
- Psoriatic arthritis – principally affects the distal interphalangeal joints. Inspect the nails for psoriatic change.
- Osteoarthritis – nodules are found, typically over the distal interphalangeal joints (Heberden's nodes) but also over the proximal finger joints (Bouchard's nodes) (Fig. 10.9).
- Trigger finger – a flexion deformity of the finger caused by obstruction of a nodular tendon within its sheath.
- Trauma – hand injuries include tendon damage and fracture. Severed extensor or flexor tendons require suturing to facilitate healing.

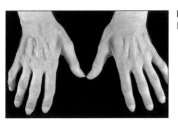

Fig. 10.10 Bilateral ulnar nerve lesions.

MUSCLE FUNCTION
Inspection
- Start with the dorsum of the hand. Wasting produces guttering between the extensor tendons, hollowing between the index finger and the thumb, and loss of the convexity of the hypothenar eminence. Look for fasciculation.
- Now, turn the hands over and inspect the palmar surfaces, concentrating particularly on the thenar eminences.

Testing power
- Start with a muscle supplied by the ulnar nerve – e.g. the first dorsal interosseous. If the muscle is weak, test other muscles supplied by the nerve, e.g. adductor pollicis and abductor digiti minimi.
- Now test the two muscles of the thenar eminence supplied solely by the median nerve – abductor digiti minimi and opponens pollicis.

Clinical application
- Carpal tunnel syndrome – weakness is confined to abductor pollicis brevis and opponens. Sensory change is often slight. Forced flexion of the wrist may trigger the patient's symptoms (Phalen's sign) and is more likely to be positive than Tinel's sign (tingling in a median distribution provoked by percussing the nerve at the wrist).
- Ulnar nerve lesion – usually occurs at the elbow, rarely distally. The affected hand muscles include the interossei, the muscles of the hypothenar eminence and the third and fourth lumbricals. Involvement of flexor carpi ulnaris and flexor digitorum profundus to the fourth and fifth digits is possible, but not inevitable, with proximal lesions (Fig. 10.10). Sensory loss occurs over the ulnar border of the hand and the ulnar 1½ digits.
- Unilateral global hand muscle weakness – the lesion is likely to be at the level of the brachial plexus or the T1 root. If the sympathetic fibres in the T1 root are involved, a Horner's syndrome appears. In the cervical rib (thoracic outlet) syndrome, a fibrous band passing from the C7 transverse process to the first rib compresses the C8 and T1 roots or the lower trunk of the brachial plexus.
- Bilateral global hand muscle weakness – causes include peripheral neuropathy, motor neuron disease and syringomyelia.

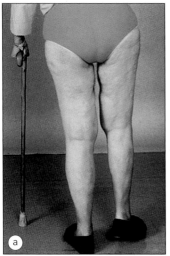 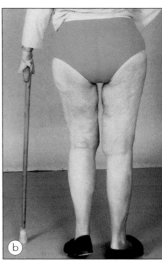

Fig. 10.11 Trendelenburg's sign. When the patient stands on the normal left leg the pelvis tilts to the left (a). When she stands on the right leg (where there was osteoarthritis at the hip) the pelvis fails to tilt to the right (b).

The hip

INSPECTION AND PALPATION
- Start with the patient standing. Look for evidence of shortening and for abnormal limb and hip postures triggered by a hip deformity.
- Ask the patient to stand, first on one leg, then the other (Trendelenburg's test) (Fig. 10.11). Normally, as the foot is lifted, the pelvis on that side tilts upwards.
- A flexion deformity of one hip can be obscured by a lumbar lordosis. In such cases, flexion of the opposite hip (with the patient lying supine) eliminates the lordosis and reveals the hip deformity (Thomas' test).
- Shortening of one leg is compensated by a scoliotic posture or by flexion of the other leg.
- An abduction deformity is compensated by flexion of the ipsilateral knee.
- An adduction deformity is compensated by flexion of the contralateral knee.

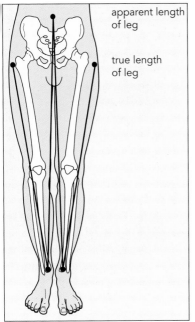

apparent length of leg

true length of leg

Fig. 10.12 True and apparent lengths of the lower limbs.

LIMB LENGTH (Fig. 10.12)

- True leg length is measured from the anterior superior iliac spine to the medial malleolus.
- Apparent length is measured from the umbilicus to the medial malleolus.
- A shortened true length suggests hip joint pathology.
- A difference in apparent lengths, with equal true lengths, indicates a pelvic tilt.

JOINT MOVEMENT

- To test hip movements alone, keep your free hand on the anterior superior iliac spine to detect any pelvic movement.
- To test flexion, bend the leg, with the knee flexed, into the abdomen.
- To test extension, stand behind the patient and draw the leg backwards until the point at which the pelvis starts to rotate.
- Internal and external rotation are tested with the hip and knee flexed to 90°.

Differential diagnosis
Hip pain

- Trauma
  - dislocation
  - fracture
- Arthritis
  - osteoarthritis
  - rheumatoid arthritis
- Slipped femoral epiphysis
- Osteochondritis (Perthe's disease)
- Infection
  - e.g. osteomyelitis

Clinical application
- Fractured neck of femur – common in the elderly. The leg becomes externally rotated, adducted and shortened.
- Dislocation – uncommon, usually posterior.
- Slipped femoral epiphysis – predominantly in adolescence. Produces pain and a limp, with limitation of flexion, abduction and medial rotation.
- Osteoarthritis – common. Joint movements are painful and restricted and eventually the limb is shortened with external rotation.

MUSCLE FUNCTION
Test hip flexors, extensors, abductors and adductors.

Clinical application
Sciatic palsy – associated with pelvic trauma, injury or infiltration by tumour. There is extensive lower limb weakness, sparing quadriceps and hip adduction. The knee reflex is intact, the ankle jerk absent.

The knee

INSPECTION AND PALPATION
- With the patient standing, look for knee deformity (genu valgum – knock-knee, or genu varum – bow-leg).
- Next test for an effusion.
- Large effusions – visibly extend down each side of the patella.
- Small effusions – perform the patella tap test. Use your left hand to force any fluid out of the suprapatellar pouch, then gently press the patella into the femur. A small effusion causes the patella to spring back.
- For smaller effusions, look for the bulge sign. Force fluid out of the suprapatellar pouch, then anchor the patella with the index finger. Now gently stroke down between the patella and the femoral condyles, first on one side, then on the other. If an effusion is present, a bulge appears on the other side of the knee.

- Palpate the joint and surrounding structures, and remember to inspect the popliteal fossa.

Clinical application
- Osteoarthritis commonly produces periarticular tenderness.
- Rheumatoid arthritis causes effusion, synovial swelling and deformity.

JOINT MOVEMENT
With the patient supine, test the range of flexion and extension.

STABILITY
- Collateral ligaments – attempt to abduct and adduct the lower leg at the knee. If there is lateral instability, record its degree.
- Cruciate ligaments – immobilise the foot, with the knee bent at a slight angle. Tense the lower leg forward and backwards. If the ligaments are lax, excessive movement occurs.

SEMILUNAR CARTILAGES
Perform McMurray's test. Bend the hip and knee to 90° then grip the heel with your right hand while pressing on the medial then lateral cartilage. Internally and externally rotate the tibia while extending the knee. If there is a cartilage tear, its engagement between the tibia and femur during the manoeuvre leads to pain, a clunking noise, and sometimes locking of the joint.

Clinical application
- Osteoarthritis – besides tenderness, leads to bony swelling around the joint and secondary quadriceps wasting.
- Trauma – meniscal tears tend to occur in young people due to a twisting injury. The medial meniscus is usually affected. Effusion appears and the knee may lock.
- Patella dislocation occurs laterally and tends to be recurrent.
- Total knee dislocation is unusual and is then usually due to a road traffic accident.

MUSCLE FUNCTION
Test the power of the quadriceps and the hamstrings.

Clinical application
- Femoral neuropathy – leads to weakness and wasting of the quadriceps, loss of the knee jerk and sensory change over the anterior thigh and medial aspect of the lower leg. Causes include thigh trauma or haemorrhage into the psoas sheath.
- L3 root syndrome – both quadriceps and hip adductors are affected, along with a depressed knee jerk and sensory change over the medial thigh and knee.

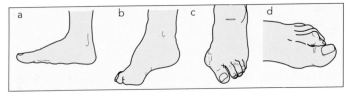

Fig. 10.13 Foot deformities. (a) Pes planus, (b) pes cavus, (c) hallux valgus and (d) hammer toe.

- Obturator palsy – causes weakness of the thigh adductors with altered sensation over the inner thigh. The problem can follow surgery, pelvic fracture or as a result of an obturator hernia.
- Meralgia paraesthetica – produces pain, tingling and numbness over the anterolateral thigh. Due to compression of the lateral cutaneous nerve of thigh in the groin.

The ankle and foot

INSPECTION AND PALPATION
- Look at the ankles from behind with the patient standing.
- Assess any deviation of the foot towards (varus) or away (valgus) from the midline.
- Assess any abnormality of the foot arch.
- Palpate the margins of the ankle joint, then the heel and Achilles tendon.
- Now assess the metatarsophalangeal joints for tenderness.

Clinical application (Fig. 10.13)
- Flat foot – the longitudinal arch of the foot is lost.
- Pes cavus – the arch of the foot is exaggerated, with hyperextension of the toes.
- Hallux valgus – abnormal adduction of the big toe at the metatarsophalangeal joint with a bursa over the head of the first metatarsal.
- Hammer toe – hyperextension at the metatarsophalangeal joint with flexion at the interphalangeal joint.

JOINT MOVEMENT
- Test plantar and dorsiflexion, and inversion and eversion.
- Test plantar and dorsiflexion of the toes.

Clinical application
- Osteoarthritis – can affect both the ankle and the foot. Involvement of the first metatarsophalangeal joint leads to hallux valgus or rigidus.

- Gout – typically affects the first metatarsophalangeal joint. Acute attacks produce a swollen, painful and red joint. In long-established cases, urate deposits appear elsewhere (e.g. the elbow and the ear).
- Rheumatoid arthritis – involves both the ankle and the foot. Various deformities develop, including subluxation of the metatarsophalangeal joints and flexion deformity of the proximal interphalangeal joints.
- Trauma – Pott's fracture is a fracture–dislocation of the ankle. Rupture of the Achilles tendon results in pain in the heel. The calf is swollen, with a palpable gap in the tendon.

MUSCLE FUNCTION
Test plantar and dorsiflexors of the ankle and toes, eversion and inversion and extensor hallucis longus.

Clinical application
- Lumbar spondylosis – commonly affects the L5 and S1 roots. With the former, weakness is often confined to extensor hallucis longus, there is no reflex change and sensory loss occurs over the medial aspect of the foot. With the latter, weakness predominates in plantar flexion, the ankle jerk is depressed and sensory loss occurs over the lateral border of the foot.
- Lateral popliteal palsy – produces weakness of dorsiflexion of the foot and toes and eversion. Sensory change is often inconspicuous. If present, it occurs over the lower shin and dorsum of the foot.

PATTERNS OF WEAKNESS IN MUSCLE DISEASE

Characteristics of primary muscle disease include:
- Symmetry.
- Proximal predominance.
- Abnormal gait with lordosis and a tendency to waddle.
- Positive Trendelenburg's sign.
- Difficulty getting up from a lying position – the patient climbs up his or her legs (Gowers' manoeuvre).
- Pseudohypertrophy of muscle due to infiltration by fat and connective tissue. The affected muscle is actually weak (Fig. 10.14).

Assessment of gait (Fig. 10.15)
- If the patient describes a gait problem, be ready to provide support.
- Observe both the pattern of leg movement and the posture of the arms.
- Observe trunk control.
- If gait appears normal, ask the patient to walk 'heel–toe'. Be ready to provide support.

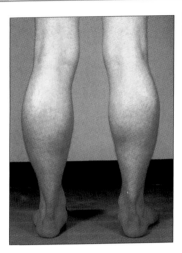

Fig. 10.14 Pseudohypertrophy of the calves.

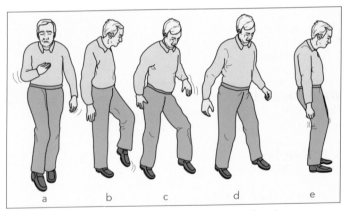

Fig. 10.15 Gait disorders. (a) Hemiplegic, (b) unilateral foot drop, (c) sensory ataxia, (d) cerebellar ataxia and (e) parkinsonism.

SPASTIC GAIT

- Hemiplegic – the arm is flexed and adducted, the leg extended. To move the leg, the patient tilts the pelvis, throwing the leg outward as well as forward (circumduction).
- Paraplegic – the whole movement is stiff, with thrusts of the trunk being used to assist locomotion.

Clinical application
- Hemiplegic gait – commonly due to cerebrovascular disease or trauma.
- Paraplegic gait – commonly due to multiple sclerosis or spinal injury.

FOOT-DROP GAIT
The patient overflexes at the knee and hip to assist foot clearance.

Clinical application
- Unilateral – lateral popiteal palsy.
- Bilateral – peripheral neuropathy.

ATAXIC GAIT
Due either to cerebellar disease or loss of sensory information from the feet (sensory ataxia).
- Cerebellar ataxia – the patient adopts a wide-based gait and lurches to one side if one cerebellar hemisphere is particularly affected.
- Sensory ataxia – the patient tends to stamp the feet to try to overcome the loss of sensory information.

Clinical application
- Cerebellar ataxia – multiple sclerosis, stroke, cerebellar degeneration, alcohol.
- Sensory ataxia – peripheral neuropathy.

WADDLING GAIT
Due to proximal lower limb weakness. The patient waddles due to a failure of the pelvis to tilt when one leg is raised from the ground.

Clinical application
Common causes – muscular dystrophy, polymyositis.

PARKINSONIAN GAIT
Shows a flexed posture with reduced arm swing and diminished stride length. There may be problems in starting, stopping and turning.

APRAXIC GAIT
A disorder of gait in which there is a particular difficulty in the organisation of walking in the absence of significant weakness, incoordination or sensory loss. The patient tends to 'freeze'.

Clinical application
The main causes are normal pressure hydrocephalus and Binswanger's encephalopathy.

HYSTERICAL GAIT

Typically bizarre and variable. Despite wild lurches, the patient seldom falls. Self-injury, however, does not exclude conversion hysteria as the cause of the gait problem.

Examination of elderly people
Bones, muscles and joints

- Muscle strength declines with age. For example, grip strength falls by approximately 50% between the ages of 25 and 80 years
- Muscle bulk declines with age, for example the small hand muscles
- Some degree of ulnar deviation at the wrists can occur with ageing
- The range of joint movement lessens with age.
- Gait becomes less certain in elderly people, with a tendency for the steps to shorten
- Elderly people tend to stand with slightly flexed hips and knees

Review
Framework for the routine examination of the musculoskeletal system

- Use GALS as a screening history and examination process
- Screening history enquires about pain or stiffness, dressing difficulty and any walking difficulty
- The screening examination assesses four areas: gait, spine, arms and legs (GALS)
- For individual joints, during a more detailed examination, a routine is followed of inspection, palpation and assessment of joint movement
- For individual muscles, the process incorporates inspection, palpation then formal testing of muscle power, using the MRC scale of 0–5
- In the lower limbs, additional stretch tests are available (straight leg raising and femoral stretch) to test for nerve root irritation in the lumbosacral region

11.
The Nervous System

HIGHER CORTICAL FUNCTION

Symptoms

MOOD
- Is the mood appropriate to the setting?
- Is the patient passive or disinterested?
- Is there anxiety or heightened arousal?

MEMORY
- Is this volunteered by the patient or by relatives?
- Does any memory loss affect recent or more remote memory?

SPEECH
- Is there word-finding difficulty (aphasia)?
- Is speech output fluent or non-fluent?
- Is there a problem with comprehension of speech, with writing (agraphia) or with reading (dyslexia)?

GEOGRAPHICAL ORIENTATION
Is it apparent that the patient has problems following familiar routes?

DRESSING
Has there been a problem with dressing, either in terms of unilateral neglect, or in terms of loss of understanding of the correct arrangement of clothes?

Examination (Fig. 11.1; Review Box p. 244)

ORIENTATION
Establish the patient's orientation in time, place and person.

MEMORY
Immediate recall
- Test digit repetition (up to seven forwards and five in reverse).

Orientation

1. What is the year, season, date, month, day? (One point for each correct answer.)
2. Where are we? Country, county, town, hospital, floor? (One point for each correct answer.

Registration

3. Name three objects, taking 1s to say each. Then ask the patient to repeat them. One point for each correct answer. Repeat the questions until the patient learns all three.

Attention and calculation

4. Serial sevens. One point for each correct answer. Stop after five answers. Alternative, spell 'world' backwards.

Recall

5. Ask for the names of the three objects asked in Question 3. One point for each correct answer.

Language

6. Point to a pencil and a watch. Have the patient name them for you. One point for each correct answer.
7. Have the patient repeat 'No, ifs, ands or buts.' One point.
8. Have the patient follow a three-stage command: 'Take the paper in your right hand, fold the paper in half, put the paper on the floor.' Three points.
9. Have the patient read and obey the following: Close your eyes. (Write this in large letters.) One point.
10. Have the patient write a sentence of his or her own choice. (The sentence must contain a subject and an object and make some sense.) Ignore spelling errors when scoring. One point.
11. Have the patient draw two intersecting pentagons with equal sides. Give one point if all the sides and angles are preserved and if the intersecting sides form a quadrangle.

Maximum score = 30 points

Fig. 11.1 The mini-mental state test.

- Serial 7s, i.e. repetitive subtraction of 7 from 100. This performance is dependent on many factors and does not specifically target patients with dementia.

Recent memory

- Enquire about three events.
- Ask the patient to memorise three objects, or a name, an address and a flower. Ten minutes later, ask them to repeat the names or objects.

- For visual memory, show the patient a drawing for 5 seconds and then, 10 seconds later, ask them to reproduce it.

Remote memory
Enquire regarding childhood, schooling, work history and relationships.

Intelligence

Test of knowledge and abstract thinking must take account of patient's social background.

LEVEL OF INFORMATION
Enquire about recent events.

CALCULATION
Give the patient simple tasks in addition, subtraction, multiplication and division.

PROVERB INTERPRETATION
Read out proverbs of increasing complexity and ask for the patient's interpretation. This assesses both general knowledge and capacity for abstract thinking.

CONSTRUCTIONAL ABILITY
Ask the patient to copy designs of increasing complexity.

GEOGRAPHICAL ORIENTATION
Problems may have been evident during history taking: assess formally by asking the patient to draw an outline of his or her country and within it place some of the major cities.

SPEECH
- Determine the patient's handedness – and not just for writing.
- There are three disorders of speech – dysarthria, dysphonia and dysphasia.

Dysarthria
A defect of articulation. Language use is normal.

Dysphonia
A defect of volume, typically the consequence of diaphragmatic, respiratory muscle or vocal cord dysfunction.

Dysphasia
A defect of language function in which there is either abnormal comprehension, or production, of speech, or both. Speech lacks grammatical content, shows word-finding difficulty and contains word substitutions (paraphasias).

ASSESSMENT OF DYSPHASIA

Fluency

- Assess the amount of speech produced in a given period of time.
- Ask the patient to name as many objects as possible in a particular category (e.g. fruits) in a set period of time.

Questions to ask
Assessment of dysphasia

- What is the patient's handedness?
- Is the speech fluent or not?
- What is the level of comprehension?
- Can the patient repeat words or phrases?
- Can the patient name objects?

Comprehension

Ask questions of increasing complexity, although still answerable by a yes or no response

Repetition

Ask the patient to repeat simple words then sentences of increasing complexity.

Naming

Ask the patient to name a succession of dissimilar objects.

READING

When assessing reading capacity, take account of the patient's education.

WRITING

Test writing by asking the patient to write first simple words then sentences to dictation. All aphasic patients have writing difficulty (agraphia).

PRAXIS

Apraxia is a disorder of skilled movement (whether of the face, tongue or limb) which is not attributable to weakness, incoordination, sensory loss or a failure to comprehend the command:

- Ideomotor apraxia – a defect for a single skilled task
- Ideational apraxia – a failure to perform a more complex sequence of skilled activity.

To assess, start by asking the patient to carry out a particular task. If that fails, ask the patient to copy your own movement and, if still unsuccessful, provide an object (for example, a screwdriver) and ask for a demonstration of its use. A more complex sequence is tested by asking the patient to go through a sequence of related movements.

RIGHT–LEFT ORIENTATION
Start with simple commands, then increase their complexity. A proportion of normal individuals have some problem with right–left orientation.

AGNOSIA
Visual agnosia – patients are unable to recognise objects, despite intact vision and speech capacity.

Primitive reflexes

A number of reflexes may emerge as the result of the disorders affecting higher cortical function.

GLABELLAR TAP
Tap your index finger repetitively on the patient's glabella. The blink response should inhibit after three to four taps. The response fails to inhibit in Parkinson's and Alzheimer's disease.

PALMOMENTAL REFLEX
Apply firm and fairly sharp pressure to the palm alongside the thenar eminence. A positive response results in contraction of the ipsilateral mentalis with puckering of the chin.

POUT AND SUCKLING REFLEXES
A positive pout response consists of protrusion of the lips when they are lightly tapped. A positive suckling reflex consists of a suckling action of the lips when the angle of the mouth is stimulated.

GRASP REFLEX
Elicited by stroking firmly across the palmar surface of the hand from the radial to the ulnar border. In a positive response, the examiner's hand is gripped by the patient's fingers, making release difficult or impossible. A foot grasp reflex is elicited by stroking the sole of the foot towards the toes with the handle of a patellar hammer. A positive response results in flexion of the toes with grasping of the hammer (Fig. 11.2).

Clinical application

DEMENTIA
Commonest causes are Alzheimer's disease, Lewy body dementia and cerebrovascular disease.

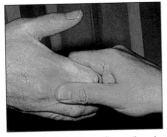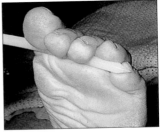

Fig. 11.2 Primitive reflexes (hand and foot grasp).

AMNESIA

Damage to the limbic system leads to failure to learn new memories (antegrade amnesia) plus loss of memory for recent events (retrograde amnesia).

 Differential diagnosis
Disorders of higher cortical function and speech

- Dementia
  - Alzheimer's disease
- Amnesia
  - postherpes simplex encephalitis
- Dysarthria
  - Brainstem stroke
- Dysphonia
  - Myasthenia gravis
- Dysphasia
  - Broca, Wernicke type
- Apraxia
  - corpus callosum lesions
- Grasp reflex
  - frontal lobe tumour

DYSCALCULIA

Occurs with unilateral or bilateral hemisphere lesions.

CONSTRUCTIONAL APRAXIA AND GEOGRAPHICAL DISORIENTATION

Tend to be associated with non-dominant parietal lesions.

DYSARTHRIA

- Bulbar palsy — combined weakness of lips, tongue and palate.
- Pseudobulbar palsy — the result of bilateral damage to the corticobulbar projections. Speech is hesitant and has an explosive, strangulated quality.

- Vocal cord paralysis – unilateral paralysis results in hoarse speech of reduced volume. With bilateral lesions, speech is virtually lost.
- Cerebellar lesions – loss of speech rhythm with fluctuation in volume and inflexion. Slurring and staccato elements are found.

DYSPHONIA

Frequently non-organic. In spastic dysphonia, a form of dystonia, inappropriate muscle contraction, particularly of the larynx, produces strained and strangulated speech.

DYSPHASIA

Non-fluent speech is associated with anterior hemisphere lesions and fluent speech with posterior hemisphere lesions.

- Broca's aphasia – non-fluent and usually dysarthric. Comprehension largely intact. Naming errors occur.
- Transcortical motor aphasia – similar to Broca's, but repetition is retained. The pathology is located above or anterior to Broca's area.
- Wernicke's aphasia – fluent, easily articulated speech but frequent paraphasias and meaning is largely lost. Comprehension and repetition severely impaired.
- Conduction aphasia – fluent, though less so than Wernicke's. Frequent interruptions to speech rhythm occur but without dysarthria. Naming is impaired but comprehension good. Repetition is severely abnormal.
- Transcortical sensory aphasia – fluent but frequently interrupted by words or phrases initiated by the examiner (echolalia). Despite this, comprehension is severely impaired.
- Anomic aphasia – fluent and interrupted more by pauses than by paraphasic substitutions. It is often the final stage of recovery from other forms of aphasia.
- Global aphasia – all aspects of speech function are affected. Output is non-fluent and comprehension, repetition and naming are all affected, often severely.

DYSLEXIA AND ALEXIA

- Dyslexia – developmental reading disorder
- Alexia – acquired reading disorder resulting from brain damage.

AGRAPHIA

Nearly all aphasic patients have agraphia, but many patients with agraphia are not aphasic.

APRAXIA

- The pathway for performing a skilled task to command begins in the auditory association cortex of the dominant hemisphere and then passes to the parietal association cortex, subsequently forwards to the premotor cortex and finally the motor cortex itself.

• Interruption of this pathway at any point results in an ideomotor apraxia affecting both the dominant and non-dominant hands.

RIGHT–LEFT DISORIENTATION
Usually the result of a posteriorly place dominant hemisphere lesion.

VISUAL AGNOSIA
• One type is caused by a disconnection between the visual cortex and the speech area.
• Another type is associated with loss of object recognition, which can be overcome if the patient handles the object.

PRIMITIVE REFLEXES
• The palmomental reflex is found bilaterally in some normal individuals. A unilateral reflex suggests a contralateral frontal lobe lesion.
• Snout and suckling reflexes are found in patients with diffuse bilateral hemisphere disease.
• Bilateral grasp reflexes are of limited localising value, but a unilateral reflex is associated with contralateral frontal lobe lesions.
• A foot grasp or tonic plantar reflex can be an early sign of a frontal lobe lesion.

THE PSYCHIATRIC ASSESSMENT

Make sure that the patient understands who you are, and the purpose of the interview. Privacy is particularly important when sensitive issues are being explored. To begin with, avoid making notes, as this can detract from the relationship you are trying to establish with the patient. During this preliminary phase, observation of the patient's posture, gestures and facial expression may provide information regarding mood and feeling. The depressed patient appears apathetic, has little expression and may well be reluctant to discuss the history. The agitated patient is restless.

History of present condition

This proceeds in much the same way as history-taking from a patient with a physical complaint. Indeed, physical symptoms often predominate in those individuals with a primary psychiatric illness. Try to establish when the patient last felt well, as a means of determining the overall length of the history and as a means then of establishing the chronological order of subsequent symptoms. If necessary interrupt the patient if he or she digress into other areas, for example current social issues, although making clear that you are interested in these issues, and will wish to return to them later. Sometimes directive questions are needed to focus the patient's attention on a particular symptom, for example headache, in order to explore that symptom in greater detail. As the history proceeds, open questions will be partly replaced by closed questions, answerable by a simple yes or no response. Sometimes signs of emotional distress may appear as certain issues are covered. Rather than ignoring these, gently probe them, even if this temporarily disturbs the course of the history.

Quite often, patients only indirectly refer to stressful issues by giving oblique reference to them in the course of describing their physical symptoms. Try to pick up the cues and develop the relevant issue. Failure to detect them may well deter the patient from discussing them further.

Many symptoms are common to both physical and psychiatric illness but others are more specifically within the territory of psychiatry.

Specific symptoms

MOOD

Enquire whether the patient, or a relative, has noticed any mood change. A particularly valuable question when screening for depression is whether the individual has lost pleasure in normal activities (anhedonia). Supplementary to this will be enquiries regarding sleep pattern, loss of libido and suicidal ideation. Sometimes the patient denies flattening of mood, when that is all too evident from the interview. Such discrepancies should be carefully recorded.

Patients will usually complain of anxiety but sometimes its somatic manifestations, for example palpitations, sweating and tremulousness, predominate. The anxiety may be chronic and spontaneous or be triggered acutely by a specific stimulus – phobic anxiety.

Patients seldom complain of euphoria – a feeling of limitless physical and mental energy. There is likely to be a pressurised, manic quality to the patient's conversation, coupled with physical restlessness.

Questions to ask
Psychiatric assessment

- Do you feel unduly anxious or depressed?
- Do you repeat certain tasks over and over again?
- Do you feel people are against you?
- Have you heard or seen things that are not there?
- Do you ever lose the sense of yourself or your environment?

ABNORMAL THOUGHTS

These will be elicited only by sensitive questioning. The patient can be understandably reluctant to reveal certain abnormal thoughts. It may be apparent from the interview that the patient's thought pattern is difficult to follow or that abnormal thoughts have pervaded the conversation. Ask the patient about paranoid ideas, in other words, whether they feel people are against them. Ask whether certain thoughts or ideas regularly intrude into their thinking, or whether they believe their thoughts are being interfered with or influenced by external agencies. Thought disorders include delusions and obsessiveness.

Delusions

These are beliefs that can be demonstrated to be incorrect but to which the individual still adheres. Members of the Flat Earth Society are deluded. Often there is an element of reference, in other words that actions or words are directed specifically at that individual even if they appear on a global platform, for example television. Paranoid delusions contain a persecutory element. Delusions of worthlessness are particularly associated with depressive illness.

	Symptoms and signs

Somatic and psychic symptoms of anxiety and depression

	Anxiety	**Depression**
Somatic	Palpitations	Altered appetite
	Tremor	Constipation
	Breathlessness	Headache
	Dizziness	Bodily fatigue
	Fatigue	Tiredness
	Diarrhoea	
	Sweating	
Psychic	Feelings of tension	Apathy
	Irritability	Poor concentration
	Difficulty sleeping	Early morning waking
	Fear	Diurnal mood swing
	Depersonalisation	Retardation
		Guilt

Obsession

These are recurrent thoughts which often result in the performance of repetitive acts (compulsion). The patient is aware that they are inappropriate but cannot resist returning to them or acting upon them. Examples of obsessional thought include convictions that a particular individual is antagonistic or that a spouse is unfaithful.

ABNORMAL PERCEPTIONS

These are auditory or visual phenomena of which other individuals are not aware.

Hallucinations are experiences that have no objective equivalent to explain them. They are predominantly visual or auditory but can occur in other forms, for example, of smell or taste in patients with complex partial seizures. *Visual hallucinations* can be unformed, for example an ill-defined pattern of lights, or formed, the individual then describing people or animals, often of a frightening aspect. Visual hallucinations are more often a feature of an organic brain syndrome (e.g. delirium tremens or an adverse drug reaction) than a functional psychosis, e.g. schizophrenia. *Auditory hallucinations* are also either unformed or formed. They are found more often in the functional psychoses than in organic brain disease. The voices can take on a persecutory quality in schizophrenia and an accusatory element in depression. In *déjà* and *jamais vu*, intense feelings of a relived experience or a sensation of strangeness in familiar surroundings occur, respectively. Both can be a feature of everyday life but when pathological are usually epileptic. *Illusions* are misinterpretation of an external reality – all of us have this when watching a magician at work. In *depersonalisation*, the individual feels a detachment from the normal sense of self, in *derealisation* a detachment from the external world. Both occur in neurotic illnesses but also, periodically in normal individuals.

The assessment of higher cortical function has already been discussed. It is necessary to distinguish cognitive impairment due to dementia, from cognitive impairment due to delirium. In the latter there is clouding of consciousness, usually manifested as reduced awareness of, or response to, the environment.

The family history

Begin by obtaining details of the patient's father and mother, in terms of their current age (or age at death), their own quality of health, whether they had any history of psychiatric disorder and the quality of the patient's relationship with them. Ask similar questions about the patient's siblings. Questions regarding the patient's own children are usually included in the personal history. Genetic factors are particularly strong in schizophrenic and manic–depressive psychosis.

The personal history

CHILDHOOD

It is unlikely that the patient will have accurate details of birth or early development unless there were particular problems with them. A direct question to the patient regarding whether he or she was happy or unhappy in childhood is useful. Some 'happy' responses turn out to be rather less so with further delving. If there is an expression of remembered unhappiness, explore it further in terms of relationships with parents and any physical illness.

SCHOOLING AND FURTHER EDUCATION

Establishing the details of this is helpful in forming an assessment of the patient's premorbid intelligence. At the same time enquire about friendships or a tendency to isolation and about teasing or bullying.

SEXUAL DEVELOPMENT

For female patients, enquire about the age of the menarche and how they attuned to adolescence in terms of menstruation and sexuality. For men, discussion should include whether their sexuality could be discussed in the home and how they acquired their sexual experience. Further issues relating to sexual development, for example homosexual experiences, are best left, at this stage, to the patient to raise.

MARITAL HISTORY

An overall outline here includes the age of the spouse, when the marriage occurred, the overall quality of the relationship, the state of the sexual relationship and details of any children.

OCCUPATIONAL HISTORY

Ask how many jobs the patient has had, reasons for leaving previous posts, the quality of relationship in the work place and the level of job satisfaction. If there has been one or more periods of unemployment, explore what affect this has had on the patient's overall welfare.

PAST MEDICAL HISTORY

This follows the usual pattern, and includes history of physical and mental illnesses if these have occurred.

DRUG HISTORY

Determine alcohol consumption, but be aware of the possibility that the figure does not correspond to actual intake. Features suggesting alcohol dependency include early morning drinking, morning vomiting, taking a drink before an interview, erratic work attendance and drinking in isolation. Ask about narcotic exposure, the use of softer drugs such as cannabis and exposure to tranquilisers. If the patient is using codeine derivatives, ascertain for what purpose and the dosage.

PERSONALITY PROFILE

Evidence suggesting changing personality and mood is often better provided by colleagues, relatives or friends than by the patient. Questionnaires exist for the assessment of personality but even without them the patient's attitude and behaviour, in terms of work and social relationships, personal ambitions, drive, level of independence and authority and response to stress, will indicate their maturity.

THE CRANIAL NERVES

First cranial nerve (olfactory)

EXAMINATION

Apply a smell to each nostril, using a squeeze bottle. Ask the patient to identify the smell or describe its characteristics.

Symptoms and signs
Disturbances of olfaction

- Hyposmia – partial loss
- Anosmia – total loss
- Dyosmia – distorted smell
- Hyperosmia – exaggerated sensitivity

CLINICAL APPLICATION

- Commonly disturbed by upper respiratory tract infection or local nasal pathology.
- Smell sensitivity is reduced in dementia and Parkinson's disease.
- Olfactory nerve compression results in loss of smell.
- Olfactory hallucinations occur in complex partial seizures.

Second cranial nerve (optic)

EXAMINATION
Visual acuity

- For distance vision, use a Snellen chart at 6 metres from the patient. A visual acuity of 6/18 means the patient, at 6 metres, can only read the line that someone with normal vision could read at 18 metres. Make sure the patients use their glasses if they need them for distance vision. A visual acuity of less than 1/60 can be recorded as counting fingers (CF), hand movements (HM), perception of light (PL) or no perception of light (NPL).
- For near vision, uses standard test types.

Colour vision

For screening purposes, use Ishihara test plates, testing each eye separately. Ask whether the patient is aware of having a congenital colour vision defect.

Visual fields

- Finger movements or a red pin can be used for testing the peripheral fields, but only a red pin for the central field.

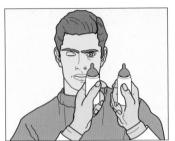

Fig. 11.3 Comparison of colour sensitivity between central and peripheral field. In this patient with a central scotoma, the red object appears brown in the central field.

- Sit approximately 1 metre from the patient. Test each eye separately, comparing the patient's field with your own. For the peripheral field, bring the target object in within the four separate quadrants of the visual field. If a red target is used, ask the patient to identify when he or she can first see the target as red. If individual half fields are full then the target object (in the form of moving fingers) should be presented in both peripheral fields simultaneously.
- Before assessing the central field, map the patient's blind spot, simply to confirm that the patient is cooperating (in terms of fixation) with the examination. Again ask the patient if he or she can identify the object as red, rather than just seeing it (Fig. 11.3).

Fundoscopy
Preferably performed in a darkened room. Ask the patient to fixate on a distant target. If severely myopic, it sometimes helps to perform fundoscopy with the patient wearing their glasses. Look for:

- The optic disc – its size, shape, colour and clarity.
- The arteries – narrower than the veins and of a brighter colour.
- The veins – particularly look for pulsation of the veins in the region of the optic disc. Retinal venous pulsation (present in about 80% of normal individuals) is lost when CSF pressure exceeds 200 mm H_2O.
- The fundus – describe any abnormal pigmentation, haemorrhages or exudates. Use a clock-face terminology to aid description, e.g. one flame-shaped haemorrhage at 3 o'clock, 1 disc diameter from the disc.

CLINICAL APPLICATION
Optic atrophy
Occurs with any process that damages the ganglion cells or the axons between the retinal nerve fibre layer and the lateral geniculate body. Pallor of the disc follows, often predominating in the temporal aspect.

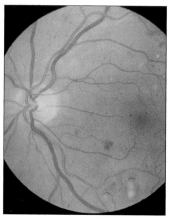

Fig. 11.4 Diabetic retinopathy. Microaneurysms, haemorrhages, exudates and cotton wool spots.

Papilloedema

Usually bilateral, although sometimes asymmetrical. Successively there is swelling of the nerve fibre layers (best seen with a red-free light), hyperaemia of the disc with loss of its definition and the disappearance of retinal venous pulsation. Eventually there is engorgement of the retinal veins, flame-shaped haemorrhages and cotton wool spots (the last due to retinal infarction). Visual field changes include enlarged blind spots and arcuate defects. Peripheral constriction is a late complication.

Retinal vascular disease

- Central retinal artery occlusion – pallor of the retina with a cherry red spot at the macula. The optic disc is first swollen then pale.
- Central retinal vein occlusion – swelling of the optic disc with dilatation of the retinal veins and haemorrhages.
- Hypertensive retinopathy – initially, variation in calibre of the retinal arteries. Later haemorrhages and cotton wool spots, and finally papilloedema (malignant or accelerated hypertension).
- Diabetic retinopathy – initially produces changes in the microcirculation leading to microaneurysms. Subsequently, haemorrhages, exudates and cotton wool spots appear. Additional features include macular oedema and infarction and new vessel formation (Fig. 11.4).

Glaucoma

Can occur in a primary form or secondary to various ocular pathologies. Changes in the optic disc include enlargement of the physiological cup. Retinal nerve fibre atrophy develops, producing arcuate field defects.

> **Symptoms and signs**
> **Visual field defects**

Absolute central scotoma	Area around fixation in which there is no appreciation of the visual stimulus
Relative central scotoma	Area in which an object is detected but its colour is reduced (desaturated)
Centrocaecal scotoma	A field defect extending from fixation towards the blind spot
Bitemporal hemianopia	Involvement of the temporal halves of both fields
Homonymous hemianopia	Involvement of the temporal half of one field and the nasal half of the other

Optic nerve disease
- The visual defect is monocular and central (central scotoma).
- Visual acuity is reduced along with colour vision.
- There is an afferent pupillary defect.

Chiasmatic lesions
Typically due to a pituitary tumour, craniopharyngioma or meningioma. The resulting field defect is a bitemporal hemianopia, typically asymmetric.

Optic tract and lateral geniculate body lesions
Uncommon. Produce incongruous (i.e. non-matching) homonymous hemianopias

Optic radiation and occipital cortex lesions
Produce homonymous defects which become increasingly congruous the more posterior the lesion. Occipital lobe lesions produce congruous defects that can be total, quadrantic or scotomatous. An isolated homonymous hemianopia is usually due to vascular disease affecting the occipital lobe.

Third, Fourth and Sixth cranial nerves (oculomotor, trochlear and abducens)

SYMPTOMS
- Ptosis – discover whether the problem is unilateral or bilateral and whether it fluctuates.

Questions to ask
Diplopia

- Is the diplopia relieved by covering one or other eye?
- Is it vertical, horizontal or oblique?
- Does it increase in one direction of gaze?
- Is it constant or fluctuant?

- Diplopia – a number of questions help to discover the underlying mechanism.

EXAMINATION
Inspection of the eyelids and pupils
- Look for ptosis and assess its fatiguability.
- Assess the pupils for size, symmetry and regularity. A slight difference in pupil size of up to 2 mm is seen in some 20% of the population (physiological anisocoria).

Pupillary light response
Ask the patient to focus on a distant object and perform the examination in a darkened room. Use a bright pencil torch. To detect an afferent pupillary defect, swing the torch from one eye to the other, while observing only the illuminated pupil.

Near reaction
There is no point in testing the near reaction if the light response is normal. Otherwise, observe the pupils as the patient fixates on a target that approaches their eyes.

INSPECTION OF EYE MOVEMENTS
Conjugate eye movements
- Pursuit – ask the patient to follow a slowly moving target, first in the horizontal then in the vertical plane.
- Saccades – ask the patient to rapidly refixate between two targets.

Doll's head manoeuvre (oculocephalic reflex)
If the eyes have failed to respond to a saccadic or pursuit movement, ask the patient to fixate on your eyes, grasp the patient's head and rotate it, first horizontally then vertically. An intact response (a measure of vestibular function) allows the patient's eyes to remain fixed on your own.

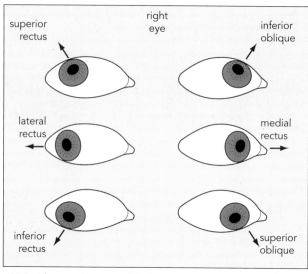

Fig. 11.5 The muscles responsible for eye movements in particular directions.

Testing individual eye muscles (Fig. 11.5)

- In strabismus, or squint, the axes of the eyes are no longer parallel.
- Concomitant squint – the angle of deviation of the two eyes remains constant. Usually congenital, and diplopia is generally absent.
- Incomitant squint – the angle of deviation varies. Usually acquired as the result of paralysis of one or more of the extraocular muscles.
- Now ask the patient to look in the six directions illustrated. The diplopia will be maximal in the direction of action of the paralysed muscle. Horizontal diplopia indicates weakness of the medial or lateral rectus. Vertical (oblique) diplopia incriminates one of the other muscles. The false image (appears indistinct or blurred) is peripheral to the true image and disappears when the eye containing the paralysed muscle is covered.
- Observe whether the patient has an abnormal head tilt as a compensation for the diplopia.

Nystagmus

Define the characteristics of any nystagmus:

- Jerk (phases of unequal velocity) or pendular (phases of equal velocity)
- Amplitude (fine, medium or coarse)
- Persistence

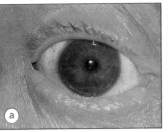 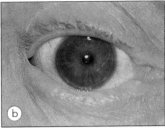

Fig. 11.6 Horner's syndrome. Before (a) and after (b) instillation of cocaine.

- Direction of gaze in which it occurs
- Horizontal, rotatory, vertical or mixed. First degree jerk nystagmus to the left has a fast phase to the left on left lateral gaze. In second and third degree nystagmus to the left, the nystagmus is present on forward gaze and to the right, respectively.

Optokinetic nystagmus

Assessed by asking the patient to observe a rotating drum, first in the horizontal then in the vertical plane. The drum is painted with vertical lines. As the patient watches the drum, a pursuit movement in the direction of the rotation is followed by a saccade, returning the eyes to the midposition.

CLINICAL APPLICATION: THE PUPIL

Horner's syndrome

- Results from interruption of sympathetic fibres to the eye.
- Combines meiosis and narrowing of the palpebral fissure due to mild ptosis of the upper lid and elevation of the lower lid.
- Enophthalmos is not confirmed by formal measurement.
- The distribution of sweating loss on the face depends on the site of the lesion
- To confirm the diagnosis, instil 4% cocaine into each eye: the normal pupil dilates, the affected pupil fails to do so (Fig. 11.6).

Tonic pupil syndrome

- Usually unilateral.
- The affected pupil is dilated but becomes smaller with time.
- The light response is absent or markedly depressed. In a darkened room, the affected pupil becomes smaller due to a failure of reflex dilatation.
- The near reaction is delayed but may eventually exceed that of the normal pupil.
- Relaxation of the near reaction is also delayed, so that for a period the affected pupil is now smaller.

- There is sometimes an associated depression of the deep tendon reflexes (Holmes–Adie syndrome).

Argyll Robertson pupil
- Miosed and often irregular pupil with evidence of iris atrophy.
- The light response is diminished or absent compared to the near reaction (light–near dissociation).
- When complete, pathognomonic of neurosyphilis.

Relative afferent pupillary defect
- Due to a lesion of the afferent light reflex pathway between the retina and the lateral geniculate body.
- Not found with disease of the lens or vitreous.
- Using the swinging light test, the affected pupil dilates as the torch swings on to it from the unaffected pupil.

CLINICAL APPLICATION: DISORDERS OF EYE MOVEMENT
Gaze paresis
- Acute frontal lobe lesion – contralateral horizontal saccades are depressed or absent and there is limb paresis ipsilateral to the gaze palsy. Pursuit and oculocephalic movements are spared. Saccades return later, then initiated by the contralateral frontal lobe.

Differential diagnosis
The pupil and eye movements

Pupillary syndromes
- Horner's
- Tonic pupil
- Argyll Robertson pupil
- Relative afferent pupillary defect

Eye movement disorders
- Gaze paresis
- Internuclear ophthalmoplegia
- One-and-a-half syndrome
- Abducens, trochlear and oculomotor nerve palsies

Nystagmus
- Congenital
- Vestibular
- Gaze-evoked
- Downbeat
- Convergence–retractory

- Paramedian pontine reticular formation lesion – ipsilateral gaze paresis for both saccades and pursuit movements.
- Posterior hemisphere lesions produce an ipsilateral pursuit paresis associated with a contralateral homonymous hemianopia.
- The dorsal midbrain syndrome (Parinaud) produces a paresis of upward saccades initially with relative preservation of pursuit. In addition there is convergence–retractory nystagmus and dilated, light–dissociated pupils.

Other saccadic and pursuit movement disorders
- Saccadic slowing is found in both Parkinson's and Huntington's disease, accompanied by disorganized pursuit.
- Progressive supranuclear palsy produces failure of downward saccades and pursuit, followed by involvement of upward and, finally, horizontal movements. Doll's head movements are spared until the final stages.

Internuclear ophthalmoplegia (INO)
- A lesion of the medial longitudinal fasciculus leads to slowing or failure of medial rectus contraction during lateral gaze.
- There is usually nystagmus in the abducting eye.
- Bilateral INO is accompanied by vertical nystagmus on up gaze.

The 'one-and-a-half' syndrome
Due to a lesion responsible for a unilateral INO spreading into the pontine gaze centre. The only remaining horizontal eye movement is abduction of the opposite eye.

Abducens palsy
- A lesion of the sixth nerve nucleus produces a gaze paresis.
- Isolated lateral rectus weakness is usually due to a lesion of the central or peripheral course of the sixth nerve. The eye fails to abduct.

Trochlear palsy
- Weakness of the superior oblique muscle occurs with a trochlear palsy, but is also found with myasthenia and dysthyroid eye disease.
- The head tilts to the side opposite the affected eye and the patient complains of diplopia, particularly on down gaze. There is defective depression of the adducted eye.

Oculomotor palsy
- Nuclear palsies tend to be either incomplete or complete but with pupillary sparing. A complete third nerve palsy cannot be nuclear unless there is involvement of the contralateral superior rectus.
- Peripheral palsies are commonly due to diabetes. The paresis is typically painful and pupil-sparing in about 50% of cases.

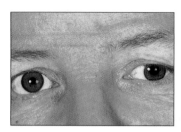

Fig. 11.7 Left third nerve paresis. The pupil is dilated.

- In a complete third nerve palsy, there is substantial ptosis and the eye is deviated laterally and slightly downwards.
- Compression of the oculomotor nerve, for example by a posterior communicating aneurysm, almost always results in pupillary dilatation (Fig. 11.7).

Combined palsies
- A cavernous sinus lesion, for example an aneurysm, is likely to affect the eye nerves in combination rather than individually. Potentially affected are the third, fourth and sixth nerves, the first and second divisions of the trigeminal nerve, and the ocular sympathetic fibres.
- A complex, mixed ophthalmoplegia, without pupillary involvement, raises the possibility of myasthenia or dysthyroid eye disease.

Nystagmus
- Pendular – usually congenital but sometimes found in brainstem vascular disease or multiple sclerosis.
- Vestibular – if peripheral, usually has both horizontal and rotatory components and is suppressed by visual fixation. If central, it is more variable and unaffected by fixation.
- Gaze-evoked – often drug-induced but also seen with disease of the cerebellum or brainstem. Vertical components indicate brainstem or cerebellar disease.
- Down-beat – when present on down and out gaze, suggestive of a foramen magnum lesion, for example a Chiari malformation.
- End-point – occurs as a physiological phenomenon at the extremes of lateral gaze and may be asymmetric.

Fifth cranial nerve (trigeminal)

EXAMINATION
Sensation
Test light touch and pin prick in all three divisions of the nerve. Remember that the third division does not extend to the angle of the jaw.

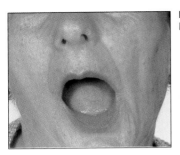

Fig. 11.8 Left trigeminal nerve lesion. Jaw deviation to the left.

Corneal response

Lightly touch the cornea with a wisp of cotton wool. Assess the ipsilateral and contralateral blink response as well as the subjective response.

Motor

Look for muscle wasting. Wasting of the temporalis produces hollowing above the zygoma. The power of the pterygoids and of masseter and temporalis can be respectively assessed by resisting attempts at jaw opening and closing. In a unilateral trigeminal lesion, the jaw deviates to the paralysed side on opening (Fig. 11.8).

The jaw jerk

Ask the patient to open the mouth slightly. Rest your index finger on the apex of the jaw and tap it with the patellar hammer. The response, a contraction of the pterygoid muscles, varies widely in normal subjects.

CLINICAL APPLICATION

- Altered motor function usually accompanies sensory loss where there is compression of the trigeminal nerve. Bilateral weakness can occur in myasthenia and Guillain–Barré syndrome. In a bilateral upper motor neuron syndrome (pseudobulbar palsy) the jaw jerk is exaggerated.
- Altered sensory function can occur in isolation with isolated trigeminal neuropathy. In spinal lesions above C2, selective loss of facial pain and temperature is possible, sometimes with an 'onion ring' distribution. Loss of facial pain and temperature occurs ipsilaterally in a lateral medullary syndrome.
- Altered corneal response may be an early or initial sign of trigeminal nerve compression.

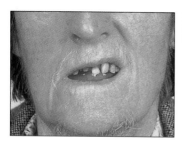

Fig. 11.9 Upper motor neuron facial weakness. The patient has been asked to bare her teeth.

Seventh cranial nerve (facial)

EXAMINATION
Although the facial nerve contains sensory fibres, they are not assessable by bedside techniques.

Motor
- Assess facial movement as the patient converses. Note any asymmetry of the forehead, eyebrows, blink or the angles of the mouth. Note whether twitching of the mouth accompanies blinking (aberrant reinnervation). Bilateral facial weakness is easily missed – the face lacks expression and appears to sag.
- Next ask the patient to elevate the eyebrows then close the eyes tightly. Try to open the eyelids by pressing them apart with your thumbs. Now ask the patient to blow out the cheeks, then purse the lips tightly together. Finally ask the patient to tighten the neck muscles in order to assess platysma.

Taste
Taste is difficult to assess by the bedside. Apply sweet (sugar), salt, bitter (quinine) and sour (vinegar) solutions to the anterior two-thirds of the tongue, first on one side, then the other. The mouth should be washed out with distilled water between applications.

CLINICAL APPLICATION
Upper motor neuron facial weakness
There is minimal asymmetry of frontalis contraction on the two sides but substantial asymmetry of the lower face (Fig. 11.9).

Lower motor neuron facial weakness
All the facial muscles are equally affected unless the lesion lies so distally that it involves individual branches of the nerve. Involvement of the nerve proximal to the origin of the chorda tympani will result in loss of taste over the anterior two-thirds of the tongue, while

involvement proximal to the departure of the nerve to stapedius will result in hyperacusis. Loss of lacrimation is added if the nerve is damaged at or proximal to the gasserian ganglion.

Bell's palsy

An idiopathic lower motor neuron facial weakness often preceded by pain. Recovery may result in regeneration of fibres which end in muscles not originally part of their innervation (aberrant re-innervation).

Ramsay Hunt syndrome

Due to herpetic involvement of the geniculate ganglion. A vesicular eruption can occur at various sites, including the pinna.

Facial movement disorders

- Fasciculation – virtually confined to patients with motor neuron disease.
- Myokymia – a subtle, shimmering motion of part or the whole of the facial nerve innervation, commonly due to multiple sclerosis.
- Hemifacial spasm – involuntary contraction of the orbicularis oculi, later spreading ipsilaterally to the other muscles supplied by the facial nerve. Eventually a mild facial weakness results.
- Blepharospasm – forced repetitive blinking. A form of focal dystonia.
- Tics – stereotyped facial movements, partly under voluntary control.
- Orofacial dyskinesias – involuntary semirepetitive contraction of muscles around the mouth, often with abnormal movements of the tongue.

Eighth cranial nerve (acoustic)

SYMPTOMS

- Deafness – if the patient complains of deafness, determine the mode of onset, whether progressive or static, and whether unilateral or bilateral.
- Vertigo – if the patient has vertigo, ascertain whether the symptom can be induced by certain postures or movements.

EXAMINATION

Each ear is tested separately. Ask the patient to occlude the ear not being tested by pressing on the tragus. Hearing sensitivity can be assessed by the capacity to hear a whispered sound (normally possible at least 0.8 m away), a wristwatch (possible at approximately 0.75 m) or the sound of fingers being rubbed together.

Rinne's test

Place a 512 Hz tuning fork on the mastoid process, then hold it adjacent to the pinna. Normally, air conduction is better perceived than bone conduction (Rinne positive). In perceptive deafness this discrepancy remains, but in conductive deafness it is reversed.

Weber's test

Place a 512 Hz tuning fork at the midline over the vertex or on the forehead and ask the patient whether the sound appears equally loud in each ear, or more so in one than the other. Normally, the sound is perceived equally by the two ears but is heard better by the intact ear in perceptive deafness and by the affected ear in conductive deafness.

Vestibular function

Peripheral vestibular function can be assessed using the head impulse test. The head is turned rapidly through about 15°, first to one side, then to the other, while the patient fixates on a distant target. In the presence of, say, a right peripheral vestibular lesion with loss of lateral semicircular canal function, when the head is rotated to the right, the vestibulo-ocular reflex fails and the eyes fail to remain fixed on the target. A saccadic correction is then made to bring the eyes back to the examiner, a movement that can be detected by the examiner.

If the patient complains of positional vertigo, position the patient at the edge of the examination couch, facing away from the edge, then depress the head and trunk so that the head is about 30° below the horizontal, but turned first to one side then, repeating the whole procedure, to the other. If nystagmus appears, record whether it begins immediately or after an interval, whether it persists or fatigues, and whether it reappears when the patient returns to the sitting position.

CLINICAL APPLICATION
Deafness

* Conductive deafness is usually due to debris or wax in the external auditory meatus, loss of elasticity of the ossicular chain (otosclerosis) or middle ear disease.
* Nerve deafness (perceptive, sensorineural) occurs with end-organ change (e.g. Meniéré's disease) or consequent to a disturbance of the acoustic nerve (e.g. after occlusion of the internal auditory artery).

Tinnitus

* Tinnitus occurs with cochlear disease, with compression of the auditory nerve, but, frequently, from unidentified causes.

Vertigo

Vertigo is usually the result of the disruption of either the labyrinthine system (peripheral vertigo) or the central connections of the vestibular nerve (central vertigo).

* Epidemic labyrinthitis and acute vestibular neuronitis – these diagnoses are applied to patients who give a history of acute vertigo, often with vomiting, together with ataxia and malaise.

Differential diagnosis
Deafness and vertigo

Conductive deafness
- Wax
- Otosclerosis
- Middle ear disease

Perceptive deafness
- Meniérè's disease
- Vascular event
- Acoustic neurinoma

Peripheral vertigo
- Vestibular neuronitis
- Benign positional vertigo
- Meniérè's disease

Central vertigo
- Cerebrovascular disease

- Benign positional vertigo – in this condition, patients experience attacks of vertigo, typically triggered by lying down in bed on one particular side. Tests for positional nystagmus are positive.
- Meniérè's disease – thought to be due to distension of the endolymphatic space. Paroxysms of vertigo occur together with persistent unilateral tinnitus and progressive sensorineural deafness.
- Central vertigo – tends to persist longer than peripheral vertigo and, if posture-related, is less likely to be delayed in onset or to fatigue after posture change compared with benign positional vertigo.

Ninth cranial nerve (glossopharyngeal)

EXAMINATION
- The motor component of the nerve cannot be tested because of the overlapping innervation from the vagus.
- To test the sensory component, assess the gag reflex. The procedure is uncomfortable and is performed only if there is suspicion of lower cranial nerve dysfunction. Press the end of an orange stick firmly into the tonsillar fossae in turn. Ask the patient if the sensation is equal on the two sides and observe the palatal elevation. In the presence of a glossopharyngeal lesion, the gag reflex is depressed or absent on that side.

CLINICAL APPLICATION
- Isolated lesions of the glossopharyngeal nerve are rare.
- Jugular foramen syndrome – affects the ninth, tenth and eleventh cranial nerves. Causes include nasopharyngeal carcinoma and glomus tumours.
- Chiari malformation – stretching of the ninth nerve leads to depression or loss of the gag reflex on one or both sides.

- Glossopharyngeal neuralgia – produces paroxysms of pain in the tongue, soft palate or tonsil, triggered by swallowing, chewing or protruding the tongue.

Tenth cranial nerve (vagus)

EXAMINATION

The nerve is tested by examining the movement of the uvula and posterior pharyngeal wall. In a unilateral vagal lesion, the uvula, either on phonation or after reflex stimulation, deviates to the intact side (Fig. 11.10). Bilateral vagal palsies produce severe palatal palsy with nasal regurgitation and aphonia.

D$_x$ Differential diagnosis
The tenth cranial nerve

Bilateral supranuclear palsy (pseudobulbar palsy)
- Stroke
- Motor neuron disease

Unilateral nuclear lesions
- Lateral medullary syndrome

Bilateral nuclear lesions (bulbar palsy)
- Motor neuron disease

Recurrent laryngeal palsy
- Aortic aneurysm
- Malignancy
- Thyroid surgery

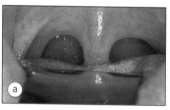

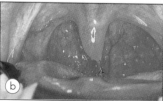

Fig. 11.10 Palsy of the left vagus. The palate deviates to the right on phonation (b).

CLINICAL APPLICATION

- A unilateral disturbance of the corticobular projection to the nucleus ambiguus is usually without effect.
- Bilateral supranuclear lesions result in a pseudobulbar palsy.
- Nuclear vagal lesions occur in polio and with lateral medullary infarction. There is ipsilateral paralysis of the palate and vocal cord.
- Recurrent laryngeal nerve palsies are common; causes include aortic aneurysm, thyroid surgery and malignant invasion. The abductors of the cord tend to be paralysed before the adductors so that the affected cord lies close to the midline. With more complete lesions, the cord lies in a position between abduction and adduction

Eleventh cranial nerve (accessory)

EXAMINATION

- Only the spinal component of the accessory nerve is assessable.
- For trapezius, ask the patient to elevate the shoulders, first without then with resistance.
- For sternomastoid, ask the patient to rotate the head against resistance.

CLINICAL APPLICATION

- Isolated lesions are rare. In the jugular foramen syndrome, the ninth, tenth and eleventh cranial nerves are affected together.
- In a hemiplegia, involvement of trapezius leads to delayed shoulder shrug on the affected side. A similar picture, but due to bradykinesia, is seen in hemiparkinsonism.
- Spasmodic torticollis is a focal dystonia affecting the sternomastoid (along with other muscles), leading to rotatory movements of the head and neck.

Twelfth cranial nerve (hypoglossal)

EXAMINATION

Inspect the tongue as it lies in the floor of the mouth. Fasciculation produces a fine shimmering motion. More coarse, involuntary movements may be seen in Parkinson's disease, Huntington's disease and orofacial dyskinesia. Assess the tongue's bulk, then ask the patient to protrude the tongue, noting any deviation from the midline, though remember that minor tongue deviation is common in normal subjects. To assess power, ask the patient to press the tongue against resistance into the cheek. Finally check the speed of lateral movement.

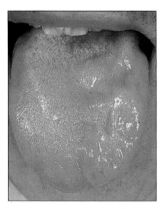

Fig. 11.11 Left hypoglossal nerve lesion.

CLINICAL APPLICATION
Unilateral lower motor neuron lesions

In a unilateral hypoglossal nerve lesion, there is focal atrophy with fasciculation and deviation of the tongue on protrusion to the paralysed side (Fig. 11.11). The problem can occur with malignant invasion of the skull base, with carotid dissection, or may be idiopathic.

Bilateral lower motor neuron lesions

These usually occur in the setting of a bulbar palsy due to motor neuron disease. The tongue is wasted and immobile. Dysphagia and dysarthria are prominent.

 Symptoms and signs
Cranial nerve examination

I Examine smell in each nostril
II Examine visual acuity, visual fields, fundi and pupillary light responses
III, IV, VI Examine eye movements and near reaction. Check for nystagmus
V Examine motor and sensory innervation, the corneal reflex and jaw jerk
VII Examine the muscles of facial expression (plus buccinator), and taste over the anterior two-thirds of the tongue
VIII Examine hearing and perform Rinne's and Weber's tests
IX Examine pain sensation in the tonsillar fossa
X Examine palatal movement and gag reflex
XI Examine sternomastoid and the upper fibres of trapezius
XII Examine tongue appearance and movements

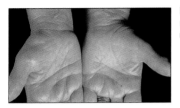

Fig. 11.12 Focal wasting of the right thenar eminence secondary to median nerve compression.

Unilateral upper motor neuron lesion

May produce slight tongue deviation to the affected side.

Bilateral upper motor neuron lesions

Part of a pseudobulbar palsy. There is dysphagia, dysarthria and emotional lability. The tongue is stiff and immobile. There is weakness of palatal elevation, combined with a brisk gag reflex and jaw jerk. The cause is usually cerebrovascular disease.

MOTOR SYSTEM

Symptoms

- When the patient describes weakness, determine its mode of onset, distribution, whether it fluctuates and whether it is associated with stiffness of the affected part.
- Although fasciculation is a physical sign, ask whether the patient has observed it. If so, check its distribution and for how long it has been apparent.
- Is the patient aware of involuntary movements? If so, determine whether they are continuous or episodic, any triggering factors and their distribution.

Examination

A detailed account of the examination of the limb muscles is given in Chapter 10.

APPEARANCE
Muscle bulk

Some thinning of the muscle bulk is common in the elderly, but not accompanied by weakness. Global loss of muscle bulk is usually due to impaired nutrition or malignancy. Focal muscle wasting (Fig. 11.12) can be prominent in the vicinity of a joint injury. Muscle hypertrophy is called pseudohypertrophy if the affected muscle is weak, the consequence of fatty infiltration.

Fasciculation

This is the spontaneous contraction of muscle fibres triggered by discharge in a single motor unit. It may be physiological (typically, then, confined to the calves), related to peripheral nerve or root dysfunction, or (particularly) a manifestation of motor neuron disease.

TONE

Ensure that the patient is relaxed. First observe any altered limb posture which might be the consequence of altered distribution of tone between antagonistic muscle groups. For screening purposes, assess flexion/extension at the elbow, pronation/supination of the forearm and flexion/extension at the knee. Use a range of speeds when displacing a joint and carry on through the whole range of movement of that joint. Take care if there is any limb or joint pain.

Spasticity

Spasticity, unless severe, is velocity dependent. In other words, it is absent at slow rates of displacement, but suddenly 'kicks in' (a 'catch') when the velocity is increased. Subsequently, the increased tone may fade as the stretch continues. In the upper limbs it predominates in flexors, and is more evident when the forearm is supinated than when it is pronated. In the lower limb it predominates in quadriceps over hamstrings.

Rigidity

Rigidity is more uniformly distributed in the limb, and is not velocity dependent. It can be accentuated by asking the patient to clench the teeth or grip the hand of the limb not being tested. At times rigidity fluctuates in a phasic manner (cogwheeling).

Gegenhalten

A more diffuse increase in tone, found in patients with an altered level of consciousness and in the presence of frontal lobe lesions.

Hypotonia

Reduced muscle tone. The limb is floppy and may show abnormal excursions when moved passively. It is found in lower motor neuron lesions and in cerebellar disease.

MUSCLE POWER

Muscle power is graded according to the MRC system of classification (see Ch. 10). In practice, grades 4 and 5 are separated by a wide range of strength requiring, as you acquire experience, the addition of grades 4+, 4++, and 5–.

For screening purposes, test deltoid, biceps, triceps, finger flexion and extension, then the first dorsal interosseous and abductor pollicis brevis in the upper limb. For the lower limb, test hip flexion and

Symptoms and signs
Definitions of paralysis

Paresis	Partial paralysis
Plegia	Complete paralysis
Monoplegia	Paralysis of one limb
Hemiplegia	Paralysis of one half of the body
Paraplegia	Paralysis of the legs
Tetraplegia	Paralysis of all four limbs

extension, knee flexion and extension, dorsi- and plantar flexion of the foot and extensor hallucis longus.

It is also worthwhile asking the patient to shrug the shoulders. A delayed elevation on one side suggests a pyramidal lesion above C2 (although the same sign can occur with an accessory nerve lesion, and with hemiparkinsonism).

If the degree of weakness fluctuates during the examination, assess fatiguability formally.

MYOTONIA
Myotonia is the result of impaired relaxation of skeletal muscle following its contraction. If the finger flexors are affected, the patient has difficulty relaxing grip. If a myotonic muscle is percussed with a patella hammer, it is likely to demonstrate a prolonged contraction, with a dimpling, for several seconds after the stimulus. The sign can be elicited in the tongue as well as in the limb muscles.

DEEP TENDON REFLEXES
Testing the reflexes assesses the integrity of the reflex arc and the supraspinal influences that affect it.

Symptoms and signs
Grading reflexes

Grade	Definition
0	Absent
±	Present with reinforcement
+	Just present
++	Brisk normal
+++	Exaggerated

UPPER LIMB

The upper limb reflexes routinely tested are the biceps, supinator and triceps.

Biceps (C5/6)

Expose the whole arm. The hands should be resting on the lower abdomen, but not crossing. For the right arm, place your left thumb or index finger on the biceps tendon, then strike your finger using a pendular motion of the hammer. If the reflex is absent, reinforce it by asking the patient to grit the teeth just before the stimulus is applied (Jendrassik manoeuvre). The left biceps tendon can be percussed only by using your left thumb with the forearm pronated.

Supinator (C5/6)

With the arms in the same position and the forearms semipronated, strike the radial margin of the forearm (interposing your finger if you wish) about 5 cm above the wrist. The response is a contraction of the brachioradialis and biceps. If the reflex is absent, or markedly depressed but finger flexion occurs, the reflex is said to be inverted. This finding (most commonly due to cervical spondylosis) is the result of depression of the reflex arc at the 5/6 level with concomitant spinal cord involvement at that level, resulting in exaggerated reflexes in lower segments.

Triceps (C6/7)

To test the right triceps reflex, bring the right arm well across the body, with the elbow flexed at about 90°, so that the triceps tendon is adequately exposed and the whole muscle visible. Strike the tendon with the patella hammer, then repeat the process on the other side.

Finger jerk (C8)

With the patient's forearm pronated, exert slight pressure on the flexed fingers with the fingers of your left hand, then strike the back of your own fingers with the patella hammer. A positive response results in brief flexion of the patient's fingertips and can be found in normal subjects. A brisk reaction suggests an upper motor neuron syndrome above that level.

LOWER LIMB
Knee (L2/3/4)

To test the knee jerks, insert your left arm underneath the patient's knees and flex them to about 60°. Tap the patellar tendons in turn. If one or other reflex is brisk, test for patellar clonus by returning the knee to the extended position, then exerting sudden but sustained downward pressure on the upper border of the patella in order to stretch the quadriceps muscle. Even two to three beats of clonus is pathological and indicates the presence of an upper motor neuron lesion.

Ankle (S1)

Abduct the relevant leg, with the hip externally rotated, the knee flexed to about 135° and the ankle flexed to just less than 90°. If hip abduction is limited, rest the leg on its fellow to gain adequate access to the Achilles tendon. If the reflex is brisk, look for ankle clonus. With the leg in the same position, forcibly dorsiflex the ankle and maintain that position. Three to four beats of symmetrical ankle clonus can occur in normal subjects, but asymmetrical or more sustained clonus is pathological.

The deep tendon reflexes are very variable in normal subjects. Some individuals have absent reflexes, even with reinforcement, although in such cases the ankle reflexes are often relatively preserved.

OTHER REFLEXES
Abdominal reflexes

Lightly draw an orange stick across the four segments of the abdomen around the umbilicus. With each stimulus, there should be a contraction of the ipsilateral abdominal wall. The abdominal responses disappear in the elderly, and are more difficult to elicit in the obese and in women who have had multiple pregnancies.

Cremasteric reflex (L1/2)

Elicited by stroking the upper inner aspect of the thigh. It leads to retraction of the ipsilateral testicle.

Plantar response (S1)

Elicited by applying firm pressure (use an orange stick) to the lateral aspect of the sole of the foot, moving from the heel to the base of the fifth toe then across the region of the head of the metatarsals. Observe any movement in the metatarsophalangeal joint of the big toe. In the presence of a pyramidal lesion, the toe dorsiflexes. Record the movement as flexor ($\downarrow$), extensor ($\uparrow$), equivocal ($\downarrow\uparrow$) or absent (o).

Anal reflex (S4/5)

Assessed by pricking the skin at the anal margin. In normal subjects, there is a brisk contraction of the anal sphincter. The tone of the anal sphincter can be assessed by inserting a finger into the anus and asking the patient to 'bear down'.

THE EXTRAPYRAMIDAL SYSTEM
Bradykinesia

- Leads to slowness of movement and its adjustment, together with a delay in the initiation of movement.
- Test for bradykinesia in the upper limbs by asking the patient to tap repetitively the back of one hand with the other, then to 'polish' the back of one hand with the other. In the lower limbs, ask the patient to tap your hand with his or her foot. Typically the movements of a

bradykinetic limb lose their amplitude and force during these procedures.

- Bradykinesia is particularly associated with Parkinson's disease.

Involuntary movement

Begin by detailing the characteristics of the movement:

- Is it present at rest, with the limb completely supported or when the limb takes up a certain posture, or when the limb is in use?
- Is the movement repetitive or random?
- Is the movement confined to a limb, a segment, half of the body or is it generalised?
- Is it mainly proximal or distal in the limb?
- Are the movements of brief duration or are they sustained?

Tremor

Tremor is a rhythmic movement that, at a particular joint, is usually confined to one plane.

Myoclonus

Myoclonus is characterised by rapid, recurring, muscle jerks.

Chorea

Choreiform movements are brief, random movements that are less shock-like than myoclonus. They can affect both the proximal and distal parts of the limb.

Athetosis

Athetoid movements are slower then chorea and become prominent during the performance of voluntary activity. They predominate distally in the hand (Fig. 11.13); the posture oscillates between hyperextension of the fingers and thumb, usually with pronation of the forearm and flexion of the digits associated with supination. In some patients, the movements are superimposed on more sustained postures.

Hemiballismus

Hemiballismus results in violent swinging movements of an ipsilateral arm and leg.

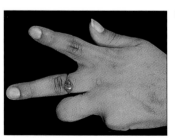

Fig. 11.13   Athetoid hand posture.

Dystonia

In dystonia, abnormal posture result from the contraction of antagonistic muscle groups.

Tics

Tics are repetitive movements that appear, at least briefly, to be under voluntary control.

Dyskinesia

Dyskinesias are brief, involuntary movements that are commonplace, around the mouth and face in the elderly (orofacial dyskinesia). Similar movements can result from dopa or phenothiazine therapy.

Myokymia

Myokymia, when confined to the eyelid and perceived as a fine twitch, is commonplace. In pathological myokymia, the movement extends to other parts of the face.

Asterixis

In certain metabolic disorders, particularly hepatic and renal failure, there is a defect of limb posture control. If the patient extends the arms and fingers, a downdrift of the fingers and hands is interrupted by a sudden upward corrective jerk.

Clinical application

MYASTHENIA

In myasthenia gravis, fatiguable weakness can affect any skeletal muscle. Diplopia and ptosis are common. The tendon reflexes are preserved. Muscle wasting is a late and inconsistent feature.

Differential diagnosis
The motor system

Upper motor neuron syndrome
- Cerebrovascular disease
- Head or spinal injury
- Tumour
- Multiple sclerosis

Lower motor neuron syndrome
- Peripheral neuropathy

- Nerve root disorder
- Motor neuron disease

Fluctuating weakness
- Myasthenia gravis

Myotonia
- Dystrophia myotonica

EXTRAPYRAMIDAL DISORDERS
Parkinson's disease
Typically produces a mixture of bradykinesia, rigidity and tremor. Postural instability is common and the neck and trunk become flexed. Arm swing is reduced when walking and turning becomes more difficult.

Multisystem atrophy
Here an extrapyramidal syndrome is accompanied by pyramidal, cerebellar and autonomic findings.

Drug-induced disorders
Many patients with rigidity and bradykinesia (akinetic–rigid syndrome) have had their symptoms induced by drugs that influence dopamine release or its receptor sites (e.g. phenothiazines).

Progressive supranuclear palsy
This condition, as well as affecting the extrapyramidal system, affects the supranuclear then nuclear pathways for eye movement, initially in the vertical plane.

MOVEMENT DISORDERS
Tremor
- Essential (familial) tremor – absent at rest. Can affect the head, neck and voice as well as the limbs. Autosomal dominant inheritance. Fifty per cent of patients find alcohol relieves the tremor.
- Parkinsonian – typically a resting tremor at 4–5 Hz, most commonly flexion/extension movements at the wrist and fingers, with pronation/supination of the forearm. It inhibits briefly with skilled movement.
- Cerebellar – typically an action tremor, increasing as the target is approached.
- Physiological – normal finding, apparent on EMG examination. Frequency around 9 Hz. Enhanced by agitation, thyrotoxicosis and sympathomimetic agents.

Myoclonus
- Palatal myoclonus – typically at 2–3 Hz. Affects the palate, larynx and face. Associated with brainstem pathology, usually vascular.
- Segmental – occurs with spinal cord disease.
- Generalised – many causes. Can be familial or acquired, e.g. subacute sclerosing panencephalitis and Creutzfeldt–Jakob disease.

Chorea
- Sydenham's (rheumatic) chorea – sometimes reappears in adult life, either spontaneously or triggered by pregnancy.
- Huntington's disease – chorea is usually a prominent feature, although not in the juvenile form.

- Other causes include thyrotoxicosis, systemic lupus erythematosus, polycythaemia and the oral contraceptive.

Hemiballismus
Usually due to a vascular lesion in the contralateral subthalamic nucleus.

Dystonia
- Torsion dystonia – a familial, generalised dystonia which may predominate in axial or limb muscles.
- Drug-induced – e.g. dopa.
- Hemi-dystonia – e.g. with contralateral thalamic lesions.
- Focal dystonias – e.g. blepharospasm, spasmodic torticollis and writer's cramp.

Symptoms and signs
Examination of the motor system

- Inspect muscle bulk and assess any fasciculation
- Examine muscle tone
- Examine power (MRC classification)
- Perform the deep tendon reflexes, the abdominal responses and the plantar responses
- Assess any involuntary movement

Myokymia
Facial myokymia is associated with brainstem tumours and multiple sclerosis.

THE CEREBELLAR SYSTEM

Symptoms

DYSARTHRIA
Patients with dysarthria have a defect of pronunciation but normal speech content.

LIMB CLUMSINESS
A unilateral cerebellar disorder results in an ipsilateral limb ataxia.

GAIT ATAXIA
If the cerebellar problem is unilateral, the patient tends to deviate to that side on walking. With involvement of midline structures, the

unsteadiness is not to a particular side, and predominates over any limb ataxia.

Examination (Review Box p. 244)

SPEECH
In cerebellar dysarthria, speech volume and pitch are erratic, so that speech rhythm is disrupted, with pauses then accelerations. When severe, the speech becomes staccato.

EYE MOVEMENTS
Examination should include pursuit and saccadic movements and assessment of any nystagmus. In cerebellar lesions, saccadic movements may under- or overshoot (hypometria and hypermetria), while pursuit movements are likely to be broken.

Symptoms and signs
Eye signs in cerebellar disease

Flocculus	Abnormal smooth pursuit + gaze-evoked nystagmus
Flocculus/nodulus	Down-beat nystagmus
Vermis/fastigial nucleus	Ocular dysmetria
Lateral zones	Ocular dysmetria + gaze-evoked nystagmus

LIMBS
- Hypotonia – see if the limb is relatively hypotonic, although this is a difficult sign to elicit
- Finger–nose test – ask the patient, using the index finger first of one hand, then the other, to touch in turn the end of his or her nose and the end of your own index finger held about 0.5 m away. In a cerebellar lesion, the relevant side or sides are ataxic, the movement becoming more disorganized as the target is approached. It may then overshoot or undershoot the target, or cannon into it.
- Alternating movements – ask the patient to tap the top then bottom of his or her outstretched hand with the palmar aspect of the fingers of the other hand. In cerebellar disease, the movement is disorganised, varying in amplitude, rhythm and force (dysdiadochokinesis).
- To assess lower limb coordination, ask the patient to slide the heel of one leg down the shin of the other. At the end of the movement, ask the patient to lift the leg in the air before setting the heel down again, just below the knee (the heel–knee–shin test). In cerebellar disease, the heel wavers along its pathway and may well descend abruptly on to the surface of the shin.

GAIT
If the lesion is unilateral, the patient will deviate to the affected side. Bilateral involvement, or relatively pure vermian involvement, produces a broad-based gait with deviation to either side and, if severe, truncal oscillation.

Clinical application
- Cerebellar hemisphere lesions – typically cerebrovascular or neoplastic. The cerebellar defect is ipsilateral.
- Midline cerebellar lesions – with involvement of the vermis or paravermis, the predominant symptom, and sign, is gait ataxia.
- Global cerebellar atrophy – often familial.

Differential diagnosis
Cerebellum

Hemisphere	**Vermis**
• Stroke	• Alcohol-related
• Primary and secondary tumours	• Hypothyroidism
• Multiple sclerosis	
• Degenerative disorders	

THE SENSORY SYSTEM

Symptoms

PAIN
- Only rarely does the quality of a pain identify its likely source.
- Causalgia is a persistent burning sensation which can follow peripheral nerve damage.
- Thalamic pain describes a persistent, unpleasant, burning or scalding discomfort, typically exacerbated by painful or tactile

Symptoms and signs
Sensory disturbances

Sensation	**Light touch**	**Pain**
Reduced	Hypaesthesia	Hypalgesia
Lost	Anaesthesia	Analgesia
Exaggerated	Hyperaesthesia	Hyperpathia
Exaggerated at normal threshold	—	Hyperalgesia

contact, which can emerge after damage to the spinothalamic tract or thalamus.

PARAESTHESIAE AND NUMBNESS

Try and determine exactly what patients mean when they use these terms. Their use may not correspond to your own.

Examination (Review Box p. 244)

- Sensory examination is difficult. The responses are largely subjective.
- Avoid fatiguing the patient by not testing sensation over a protracted period.
- If there is a complaint of reduced sensation, start testing within it, then moving out towards the zone of transition to normal sensation.

LIGHT TOUCH

- Use a wisp of cotton wool.
- Do not drag the stimulus over the skin: apply it at a single point.
- Test with the patient's eyes closed.
- In parietal lesions, the half-body supplied by the damaged cortex may fail to register a stimulus when a second stimulus is applied simultaneously to the intact side, although it does perceive the stimulus when applied in isolation (sensory suppression or extinction).

TWO-POINT DISCRIMINATION

- This is tested using a pair of compasses specifically designed for the purpose, with gradations in centimetres indicating the separation of the tips.
- In a young adult, threshold is around 3 mm on the fingertips, 1 cm on the palm and 3 cm on the sole of the feet.

PROPRIOCEPTION

- When testing proprioception, avoid pressing on the digit in such a way that the patient might appreciate the direction of movement.
- To test the terminal interphalangeal joint of the index finger, grip the sides of the digit with your own right thumb and forefinger, using your left hand to stabilise the proximal joints of the finger. If responses are inaccurate (do about six random movements), move to a proximal joint. Normally, movements can be accurately perceived which are barely visible to the naked eye.
- Active proprioception can be tested by asking the patient to locate a digit of one hand with the index finger of the other with the eyes closed. If proprioceptive loss in the hands is severe, the fingers of the outstretched hand, while the eyes remain closed, will wander in a purposeless fashion (pseudoathetosis).

- When there is substantial loss of proprioception in the feet, the patient, standing with the feet together, can retain stability with the eyes open, but loses it with the eyes closed (positive Romberg's test).

VIBRATION SENSE
- Vibrations sense is tested using a 128 Hz fork.
- To test the fingers, apply the base of the gently vibrating fork to the pad or the knuckle of the distal interphalangeal joint.
- To test the foot, start over the interphalangeal joint of the big toe.
- If vibration sense is absent distally, move proximally, but there is no point, in the lower limbs, going beyond the anterior superior iliac spines.

PAIN
- Test using a sharp pin, but not a venepuncture needle.
- Dispose of the pin as a contaminated 'sharp' as soon as you have completed testing.
- Deep pain can be tested by applying pressure to deeper structures, e.g. by pinching the tendo Achilles.

TEMPERATURE
- Generally tested by using metallic tubes containing, respectively, hot water and ice.
- Test the temperature on your own skin before examining the patient.

WEIGHT, SHAPE, SIZE AND TEXTURE
- Certain sensory modalities are worth testing if a disturbance of cortical function is suspected.
- For weight application, put an object in the patient's hand and ask them to assess its weight, comparing it with a comparable weight in the other hand.
- For shape, ask the patient to assess various coins, including whether or not the coin has a milled edge, although that introduces other sensory modalities.
- Materials, e.g. silk, linen or wool, can be used to test appreciation of texture.

Clinical application

NERVE AND ROOT DISORDERS
- Within an affected nerve or root distribution all sensory modalities will be equally affected.
- Around that area is a zone of partial loss in which light touch appreciation is more affected than pain and temperature.

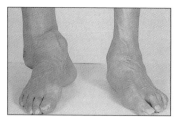

Fig. 11.14 Charcot joint. Right ankle.

- Involvement of pain fibres to the skin and joints can lead respectively, to painless skin ulceration and to severe joint derangement (Charcot joint, (Fig. 11.14)).

SPINAL CORD DISORDERS
- Transverse cord lesion – sensory level around the site of the lesion often with a small zone in which cutaneous stimulation evokes a painful reaction.
- Unilateral cord lesion (Brown-Séquard) – produces contralateral loss of pain and temperature to a level slightly below the lesion with ipsilateral weakness and depression of vibration and joint position sense.
- Central cord lesion – disrupts crossing spinothalamic fibres, leading to bilateral selective loss of pain and temperature over the affected segments (Fig. 11.15).
- Dorsal column lesion – interferes with vibration sense, proprioception and two-point discrimination. Some patients with cervical dorsal column lesions describe a shock-like sensation radiating down the spine when the neck is flexed (Lhermitte's sign).
- External compression – tends to spare the deeper fibres in the spinothalamic tract which have emanated from segments immediately below the level of compression.
- Brainstem and thalamic disorders – in the medulla, lateral lesions predominantly affect contralateral pain and temperature sensation while medial lesions disrupt sensation served by the dorsal columns. Thalamic lesions affect all sensory modalities contralaterally.

CORTICAL LESIONS
Aspect of cortical sensory function include:

- Definition of object size, weight and texture (loss of this facility = astereognosis)
- Accurate definition of site of contact of a stimulus and discrimination of single from multiple stimulation
- Joint position appreciation.

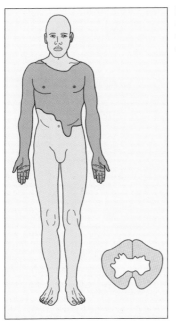

Fig. 11.15 'Cape' of selective pain and temperature loss due to a central cord lesion extending from approximately C3 to D10.

Sensory suppression is a particular feature of cortical lesions. In non-dominant parietal lesions, neglect of the contralateral limbs can be so profound that the patient denies their existence and tries to remove them as if belonging to another person.

NON-ORGANIC SENSORY LOSS

The commonest pattern of non-organic sensory loss is one in which cutaneous sensation to all modalities is affected, with little or no change in proprioception. Typically, a single limb is involved, but sometimes the problem occupies one side or the lower half of the body (Fig. 11.16).

THE UNCONSCIOUS PATIENT

Coma is usually due to:
- Extensive bilateral hemisphere disease, or
- Unilateral hemisphere mass lesion, or
- Brainstem pathology.

Mass lesions in one cerebral hemisphere affect the conscious level by herniating through the tentorial notch, with secondary compression of the brainstem. Two types of herniation occur:

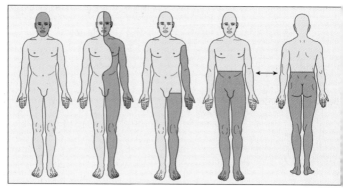

Fig. 11.16 Patterns of nonorganic sensory loss.

- Central – usually associated with slowly expanding, medially placed masses
- Uncal – in which masses in the middle cranial fossa, particularly of the temporal lobe, cause displacement of the medial aspect of the uncus over the free edge of the tentorium.

Examination

- General – check overall appearance and posture of the patient.
- Skin – carefully examine the skin for abnormal coloration, bruising and petechial haemorrhages.
- Skeletal – palpate the long bones for fractures. Inspect the skull for any swelling, and the external auditory meati for blood.
- Cardiovascular – check blood pressure, pulse and heart sounds.
- Respiratory – record the respiratory rate and rhythm and check for foetor.
- Gastro-intestinal – palpate the abdomen for organomegaly or masses.
- Level of consciousness – grade the conscious level and record the patient's Glasgow coma scale (Fig. 11.17).

Signs of meningeal irritation – look for neck stiffness and carry out Kernig's test by flexing the leg at the hip, with the knee flexed, then extending the knee. The patient may react as the knee is extended or there may be an obvious reflex spasm in the hamstrings. If the patient is deeply unconscious, these signs of meningeal irritation will disappear.

PUPILS
Use a bright pencil torch.
Make sure that drops have not been inserted and do not insert them yourself.

	Patient's response	Score	08.00	10.00	12.00
Eye opening	spontaneous	4			
	to speech	3			
	to pain	2			
	none	1			
Best verbal responses	orientated	5			
	confused	4			
	inappropriate	3			
	incomprehensible	2			
	none	1			
Best motor responses	obeying	6			
	localising	5			
	withdrawing	4			
	flexing	3			
	extending	2			
	none	1			

Fig. 11.17 Glasgow coma scale.

- Metabolic coma – the pupils usually remain reactive and symmetrical.
- Drug–induced coma – dilated pupils with atropine, amphetamines and tricyclic antidepressants. Constricted pupils with morphine.
- Structural lesions:
  Pre-tectal – mid-position fixed pupils
  Oculomotor complex – slightly irregular pupils fixed to all forms of stimulation
  Third nerve lesions – 'down and out' eye with fixed dilated pupil.
- Ocular movements – record any spontaneous movements, which can be slightly dysconjugate in unconscious patients in the absence of focal pathology of the oculomotor apparatus.

EYE MOVEMENTS

- Perform the doll's head manoeuvre. If reflex eye movements are absent, proceed to the cold caloric test by instilling 50 ml of iced water gently into one ear then the other, with the patient's head about 30° above the horizontal. If brainstem reflexes are intact, the eyes deviate to the side of the irrigated ear. For testing reflex vertical movements, the ears have to be simultaneously irrigated with cold (down-gaze) then warm (up-gaze) water.
- Frontal lobe lesion – with destructive lesions, the eyes deviate to the side of the lesion, and away from the hemiplegia.
- Brainstem lesion – if below the decussation of the supranuclear pathway for horizontal gaze, the eyes deviate toward the side of the hemiplegia.
- Upper–midbrain lesions – lead to an early failure of up-gaze.

- Pontine lesions – may produce an internuclear ophthalmoplegia, the one-and-a-half syndrome or ocular bobbing (in classical ocular bobbing, repetitive downward jerks of the eyes are succeeded by a slow upward drift).

MOTOR RESPONSES

Assessed partly by observing the patient's posture and partly by assessing response to a noxious stimulus (pressure over the sternum, a nail bed or the tendo Achilles).

- Decorticate posturing – leads to flexion and adduction of the upper limbs with extension of the lower limbs. Typically occurs with an acute vascular event affecting the cerebral hemisphere or capsule.
- Decerebrate posturing – produces extension, adduction and hyper-pronation of the upper limbs with extension of the lower limbs. Appears with midpontine lesions.

RESPIRATORY STATUS

- Cheyne–Stokes respiration – waxing and waning respiratory rate with intervening periods of apnoea seen in metabolic coma and with bilateral deep hemisphere lesions.
- Central neurogenic hyperventilation – persistently increased respiratory rate seen in midbrain/pontine lesions.
- Apneustic breathing – produces short periods of respiratory arrest on inspiration. Found in pontine lesions.
- Ataxic respiration – erratic in timing and depth, due to lesions of the medullary respiratory centre.

Clinical application

METABOLIC COMA

- Pupils usually reactive until later stages.

Differential diagnosis
Causes of coma

Metabolic
- Hypoglycaemia
- Hyperglycaemia
- Uraemia
- Hepatic encephalopathy
- Hypercapnoea
- Drugs

Structural
Hemisphere mass lesions, e.g.
- Malignant tumour
- Extradural haematoma
- Subdural haematoma
- Stroke
- Head injury

- Eye movements – eyes central and parallel apart from occasional cases showing conjugate downward deviation. Reflex movements may eventually be lost.
- Motor responses – seizures can occur, either generalised or focal. Myoclonic jerks are seen in uraemia and with hypercapnoea.
- Decorticate and decerebrate posturing are both described.
- Hemiplegia seen in hypoglycaemia and in hepatic coma.

STRUCTURAL COMA
Central herniation (due to supratentorial mass)
- Pupils – initially reactive, later, with midbrain involvement, fixed.
- Eye movements – initially loss of up-gaze. Later, horizontal movements lost.
- Motor responses – initially a contralateral hemiplegia. The unaffected side is initially decorticate then decerebrate.
- Respiration – typically initially Cheyne–Stokes; later central neurogenic hyperventilation.

Uncal herniation (due to supratentorial mass)
- Pupils – ipsilateral pupil dilates then fixes. Contralateral pupil fixed later.
- Eye movements – ipsilateral third nerve palsy; reflex eye movements in contralateral eye are initially normal, later lost.
- Motor responses – may be early ipsilateral hemiplegia; later bilateral decerebrate posturing.
- Respiration – initially no specific dysrhythmia; later central neurogenic hyperventilation; and finally ataxic respiration.

The final stages of the two types of herniation are similar.
  The clinical features of the coma associated with brainstem lesions are much more varied.

BRAIN DEATH
- The end point of many structural and metabolic insults to the brain is a state in which a deeply comatose patient maintains circulatory function providing respiration is supported.
- If brainstem functions can be shown to have ceased in such patients, there is no prospect of recovery.
- Criteria of brainstem death have been devised to assess these brainstem functions, in order to identify those patients in whom further attempts at lifesupport are of no value (Fig. 11.18).

1. *Pupillary responses*: absent using a bright pencil torch.
2. *Corneal responses*: absent.
3. *Vestibulo-ocular reflex*: tested by instilling 50 ml of ice-cold water into the external auditory meatus of one ear, then the other; there must be no response.

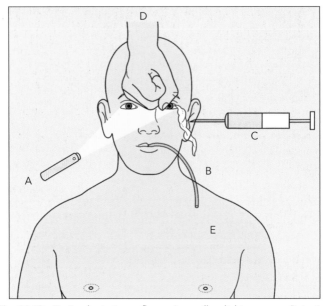

Fig. 11.18 Testing brainstem reflexes. A, pupillary light response; B, testing the corneal response; C, injection of ice-cold water to test the vestibulo-ocular reflex; D, stimulating the glabella with the knuckle; E, stimulating the trachea with a suction catheter.

4. *Motor response in cranial nerve distribution*: apply a painful stimulus to the glabella; there must be no response.
5. *Gag or tracheal response*: either stimulate the palate or pass a suction catheter into the trachea; the patient fails to respond.
6. *Respiratory reaction to hypercapnoea*: administer 95% O_2 + 5% CO_2 via the respirator until the $p\text{CO}_2$ exceeds 6 kPa; disconnect the respirator, but administer 100% O_2 through a tracheal catheter at around 6 litres per minute; there is no respiratory response to the $p\text{CO}_2$ rising above 6.7 kPa

Certain spinal reflexes can be elicited even in the presence of brain death. They include the stretch reflexes, the plantar responses and flexion of the upper or lower limb triggered by neck flexion.

Examination of elderly people
The nervous system

Primitive reflexes
- Glabellar tap – found with increasing frequency with age
- Palmomental reflex – bilateral responses found with increasing frequency with age
- Snout and suckling reflexes – seldom, particularly the latter, found in normal elderly individuals
- Grasp reflex – the presence of grasp reflexes correlates with evidence of cognitive impairment

Cranial nerve funtion
- Smell – sensitivity declines after the age of 65 years
- Eyes
  - mild ptosis common in elderly people
  - up-gaze declines with age
  - the light and accommodation responses decline with age and the pupils become more miosed
- Taste – sensitivity declines with age, with a higher threshold
- Hearing – declines with age

Motor system
- Reflexes
  - contrary to established teaching, the ankle jerks are preserved in old age
  - the abdominal responses diminish and their latency increases with age
- Movements
  - lingual–facial–buccal dyskinesias are found in elderly people without a history of neuroleptic drug exposure

Sensation
- Vibration – threshold for appreciation increases with age
- Two-point discrimination – threshold increases with age

Gait
- Becomes increasingly cautious with increasing age

Review
Assessment of higher cortical function

- Orientation
  - time, place and person
- Memory
  - immediate, short-term, remote
- Level of information
- Calculation
- Proverb interpretation
- Constructional ability

- Geographical orientation
- Speech
  - articulation, volume, fluency, comprehension, repetition, naming
- Reading and writing
- Praxis
- Right–left orientation
- Gnosis

Review
Examination of the cerebellar system

- Assess articulation
- Examine pursuit and saccadic eye movements and analyse any nystagmus
- Examine the finger–nose and heel–knee–shin tests
- Assess gait

Review
Sensory examination

- Light touch
- Two-point discrimination
- Proprioception
- Vibration sense

- Pain and temperature
- Cortical sensory function
- Sensory suppression

12.
Infants and Children

TAKING A HISTORY

In previous chapters, advice was given on how to approach patients who provide their own histories of complaints and symptoms; children come to the doctor with their parents and it is the parents who usually supply these details, although older children will often make important contributions.

Try and allow the children (including the siblings) to feel relaxed and comfortable during the consultation; this is more likely if there are a variety of toys and games lying about the room.

After the presenting complaint has been defined, information about the child's previous well-being and that of the family and their circumstances need to be recorded.

In the very young child, history-taking should include information about the pregnancy, labour and delivery as well as the condition at birth and early feeding progress, details of immunisations and a developmental history. Previous illnesses, hospital or doctor attendances as well as recent and previous medications are required in any child's history.

Include details about parents' and siblings' medical histories and make direct queries in line with the presenting problems. If an autosomally recessive condition is being considered, it may be necessary to ask if the parents are consanguineously related.

The social history is separate from but allied to the family history. It is important to understand the composition of the household in which the child lives. Include details about the parent's occupations and whoever else is helping with child care.

Child abuse is a common problem. Children can be harmed by adults in a number of different ways: emotionally, physically, neglected, sexually or, rarely, by induced illnesses and poisoning. The nature of any injury or illness in any child, from any background, must be explained satisfactorily in the history and be a plausible cause of the findings seen on examination.

THE EXAMINATION

How one approaches a child to be examined is determined by the child's age, level of development and understanding. The younger the child (except in the youngest of infants), the more imaginative one may have to be to ensure a satisfactory consultation.

Try not to allow your eye level to be higher than that of your patient. Always remember what it is like from the child's perspective, especially when being surrounded by a group of unfamiliar adults.

Whenever possible start peripherally with the hands or feet, making it clear to the child that you are a friendly doctor. Percussion is rarely a rewarding process in the very young.

Young patients should think the examination is fun: if you present yourself as playing a game, they will be relaxed and you will gain more information. Ensure your hands are clean and warm and that your stethoscope will not be too cold on the child's skin.

Avoid unpleasant procedures if at all possible (e.g. rectal examinations). It is better to have a limited but tolerable examination than to try and complete a full examination that results in an inconsolable child.

GROWTH AND DEVELOPMENT

Growth

The continuum of growth from baby to adult has been described by three main phases (Fig. 12.1):

- The infant phase: a continuation of the exponential fetal growth rate that slows down into the second year of life. The critical factors in this phase are nutrition and hormones controlling metabolism, such as insulin-like growth factors (IGF) such as IGF1.
- The childhood phase: this extends from the second to beyond the 10th year. The critical factors in this phase are the pituitary hormones (especially growth hormone).
- The adolescent (pubertal) phase: this extends from the onset of puberty until the achievement of final adult stature and fully mature reproductive capabilities. The critical factors in this phase are the sex steroids (androgens and oestrogens).

Any examination of a child is incomplete without an assessment of growth and development. It is usual to assess weight in all ages, supine length (Fig. 12.2) and head circumference in infants (under 2 years), and standing height (Fig. 12.3) in older children. Growth charts are used to help to determine the expected range at any given age.

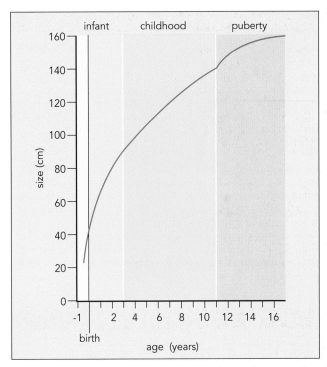

Fig. 12.1 Three phases of growth in childhood (after Professor J. Karlberg). The growth velocity varies at different ages, as result of many variable influences. Karlberg summarised the continuum into three phases, each with their own principal factors.

Development

The evaluation of a child's development is more complicated than an assessment of growth. For convenience, development is usually considered under eight main headings, which can be easily remembered as four sets of pairs

• Gross motor	Motor skills
• Fine motor	Motor skills
• Vision	Special senses
• Hearing	Special senses
• Expressive language	Communication
• Comprehension	Communication
• Social skills	Psychosocial
• Behaviour	Psychosocial

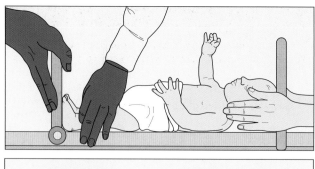

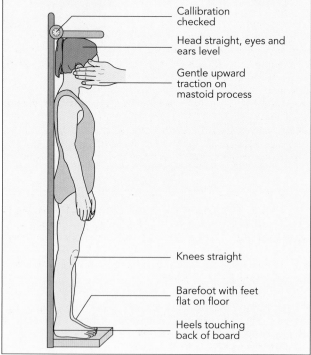

Callibration checked

Head straight, eyes and ears level

Gentle upward traction on mastoid process

Knees straight

Barefoot with feet flat on floor

Heels touching back of board

Figs. 12.2 and 12.3 Measurement of supine length and standing height. The measurement of length or height can be misleading and inaccurate unless done correctly, especially in infants.

THE NEWBORN AND VERY YOUNG BABY

Newborns and young babies are examined routinely at birth, at approximately 6 weeks of age and when receiving immunisations.

Review
Gestation and weight of gestation

- Term
  - born before 37 and 42 completed weeks gestation from last menstrual period (LMP)
- Preterm
  - born before 37 completed weeks (259 days) gestation from LMP
  - note that a preterm baby's age can be expressed as either a chronological (uncorrected) age or an age postconception (corrected); the latter is important when considering growth and development in the first 2 years
- Post-term
  - born after 42 completed weeks (294 days) gestation from LMP
- Small for gestational age or 'small for dates'
  - birth weight below 10th centile for gestational age
- Large for gestational age or 'large for dates'
  - birth weight greater than 90th centile for gestational age

---

Baby check is a system to help parents, health professionals and carers to assess the seriousness of a baby's illness. It uses 19 signs and symptoms and scores when added together give a total. The total scores correlates with the seriousness of the baby's illness.

The scoring system has been validated for use by parents, doctors and nurses in babies under 6 months old.

Total scores

0–7	Baby is only a little unwell, medical attention is not necessary.
8–12	Baby is unwell but not seriously, seek advice from doctor, health visitor or midwife.
13–19	Baby is ill, contact your doctor and arrange to be seen.
>20	Baby is seriously ill and needs to see a doctor immediately.

If the baby appears to be worse after a low score, then re-examine the baby and rescore.

1.	Unusual cry	e.g. high pitched, weak, moaning or painful	Score 2
2.	Fluids taken in previous 24 hours	Less than normal Half normal Very little	Score 2 Score 4 Score 9
3.	Vomiting	Vomiting at least half of a feed in the three previous feeds	Score 4
4.	Vomiting bile	Any green bile in vomit	Score 13
5.	Wet nappies (urine output)	Less urine than normal	Score 3
6.	Blood in nappy	Large amount of blood in nappy	Score 11
7.	Drowsiness	Occasionally drowsy Drowsy most of the time	Score 3 Score 5
8.	Floppiness	Baby seems more floppy than normal	Score 4
9.	Watching	Baby less watchful than normal	Score 2
10.	Awareness	Baby responding less than normally to the surroundings	Score 2
11.	Breathing difficulties	Minimal recession visible Obvious recession visible	Score 4 Score 15
12.	Looking pale	Baby more pale than normal, or been pale in last 24 h	Score 3
13.	Wheezing	Baby has wheezy breathing sounds	Score 2
14.	Blue nails	Apparent blue nails	Score 3
15.	Circulation	Baby's toes are white, or stay white for 3 s after squeezing	Score 3
16.	Rash	Rash over body, or raw, weeping area >5 × 5 cm	Score 4
17.	Hernia	Obvious bulge in scrotum or groin	Score 13
18.	Temperature (rectal)	Temperature is >38.3°C by rectal thermometer	Score 4
19.	Crying during checks	If baby has cried during checks (more than a grizzle)	Score 4

The very young often have nonspecific symptoms and signs even when they are seriously ill. 'Baby check' (see Box) has been validated for use by parents, hospital and community health professionals.

Doctors need to know the most important signs and symptoms of serious ill health in the very young.

Newborns and young babies can become very sick quickly. Infections should be included in the differential diagnosis of any sick baby.

Growth

Newborns tend to lose from 5 to 10% of their birth weight in the first week but then steadily gain an average of 35–30 g per day over the next 6 months. The head circumference is a valuable measurement during this period.

Development

At birth, the newborn can hear, smell, taste, feel and see (but only up to approximately 30 cm). The social smile is a very important milestone of higher cortical function. Most behaviour observed in newborns before this even is the result of responses initiated by the brainstem and spinal cord; for example, startling to sound and the primitive reflexes.

History

The feeding history is important. Any compromise in cardiorespiratory function is revealed in difficulty in taking or completing feeds. In breastfed babies, it is difficult to be certain how well the feeding is progressing because the quantities of feed are unknown. Ask the mother how often and for how long her baby breast feeds, how she feels the feeds are progressing, and whether she has any subjective feelings of let down of milk. Documented weight gain in the baby and the mother feeling that her breasts empty are helpful indicators.

Examination

You should plot the progress of weight and head circumference on a centile chart. The baby must be undressed to be fully examined.

CIRCULATION AND CARDIOVASCULAR

Auscultation of the heart sounds and listening for murmurs may be the priority before the baby cries. Inspection of the newborn's colour and perfusion is crucial. Peripheral cyanosis is common in the first days of the newborn period (acrocyanosis) because of vasoconstriction and relative polycythaemia (haemoglobin range 14.9–23.7 g/dl at birth): capillary refill time may therefore be more sluggish. Central cyanosis is best observed in the tongue. On inspection, the only signs of congenital heart disease, may be respiratory distress at rest. A pale baby may be anaemic or even hypoxic.

The rate, rhythm and character of the brachial and femoral pulses need to be assessed. Weak or absent femoral pulses may suggest coarctation of the aorta, as would four-limb blood pressure measurements demonstrating an upper limb to lower limb gradient in blood pressure. Large volume pulses are found with a patent ductus arteriosus. The precordium should be palpated and the presence of an apex beat (usually on the left) and heaves or thrills noted.

A single second heart sound may indicate pulmonary outflow obstruction. Innocent (nonpathological) systolic murmurs are common in the newborn and may be heard on day 1 in over 20% babies who have structurally normal hearts. Pansystolic and continuous murmurs are suspicious, as are ejection systolic murmurs that radiate to the back or neck. Many babies with structural congenital heart disease may not have a murmur, although they may have symptoms and other signs of cardiovascular disease.

BREATHING AND RESPIRATION

Respiratory distress is the most important observation to be made. Auscultatory signs are usually far less significant.

All babies are obligate nose-breathers during feeding and nasal obstruction may manifest as a feeding problem. Audible inspiratory stridor or a hoarse cry warrants further evaluation.

Differential diagnosis
Respiratory distress

The combination of some or all of the following:
- Tachypnoea (normal upper limit varies with age)
- Recession (includes subcostal, intercostals or tracheal tug)
- Grunting (an end-expiratory groaning noise, breathing out against partially adducted vocal cords and providing self-positive and expiratory pressure)
- Flaring of nostrils (the alae nasi are accessory muscles of respiration)
- Cyanosis (may be subclinical, so check oxygen saturation with pulse oximeter)
- Apnoea (may be how a very young baby presents with a respiratory disorder, associated with a colour change (pallor or cyanosis)
- A periodic breathing pattern may be noted in preterm or very young babies and is physiological, often with pauses of 3–5 seconds being observed (especially during sleep) without a change in colour being seen

ABDOMEN

Vomiting or 'posseting' of small quantities of milk is common but bile-stained vomiting warrants urgent assessment.

Jaundice is very common. When seen in the first 24 hours of life it is usually due to a pathological haemolytic process. A physiological jaundice is extremely common after the second day, continuing into the second week. It is usually related to breastfeeding. If jaundice is in association with pale stools, dark urine or failure to thrive, then pathological hepatic or obstructive cause is much more likely.

The palate must be inspected and palpated for clefts. The position and patency of the anus needs to be checked. While viewing the perineum, the external genitalia should be inspected. In boys, both testes should be in the scrotum. Small hydroceles are common and need no action. The penis should have a normally sited urethral orifice with a foreskin adherent to the glans. In girls there should be an introitus and a normally sized clitoris. Any ambiguity in the genitalia requires urgent assessment by a paediatric endocrinologist before sex is assigned.

The abdomen should not be distended. Divarication of the rectus abdominis muscles is common, as are umbilical hernias. The umbilical stump has usually separated by the 10th day.

A liver edge is usual palpable (approximately 1 cm below the costal margin).

Examine the hips while the nappy is off. The Ortolani and Barlow manoeuvres are used to detect abnormalities in the hip joint.

 Questions to ask
Jaundice in young babies

- Was the baby jaundiced in the first 24 hours of life?
- Was the baby still jaundiced during the third week of life?
- Is the baby well, thriving and gaining weight?
- What is the colour of the stools and the urine?

NEUROLOGY AND DEVELOPMENT

A feel of the anterior fontanelle is part of the assessment of a newborn baby. Bulging fontanelles indicate raised intracranial pressure, as in hydrocephalus, meningitis or other causes of space-occupying lesions.

Moulding or caput is common in the first 24 hours, as is a 'chignon' after a ventouse delivery. Swelling over either parietal bones is usually caused by cephalohaematomas (subperiosteal bleeds).

The best way to assess a newborn's nervous system is to observe the baby. Eliciting all the primitive reflexes is less helpful than observation. Any asymmetry of tone or movement must only be considered

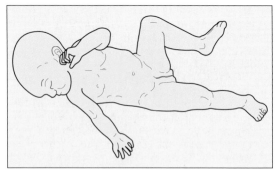

Fig. 12.4 Asymmetric tonic neck reflex (ATNR). If there is asymmetry of tone, recheck with head in the neutral midline position to avoid the influence of ATNR.

if the baby's head is in the neutral position in the midline. The asymmetric tonic neck reflex (Fig. 12.4) is a strong influence on posture and movement. The rest of the primitive reflexes may then be helpful if there are concerns about movement.

The baby should be able to fix on and follow an object through 90°. Using an ophthalmoscope, look for the presence of a red reflex in each eye. Any absent red reflex may be due to a cataract. Squints can be normal when under 8 weeks old but should diminish with age.

Young babies should startle to loud noises and should quieten to sounds that are loud and constant.

The routine neonatal examination

This examination has a number of objectives. It is a form of screening, attempting to identify congenital abnormalities that may benefit from intervention. The examination is best performed at or beyond 24 hours of age.

Examine neonates in front of the parents. As neonates are 'new and untested', this examination, more than any other at a later date, is more likely to reveal congenital abnormalities. Single minor congenital abnormalities occur with a frequency of up to 14% of live births. Severe and lethal congenital abnormalities are seen in about 1.5% of live births. Examine the undressed baby in a warm environment (Figs 12.5, 12.6).

OLDER BABIES AND TODDLERS

The term 'infant' has been used previously to describe children under 2 years of age. We prefer to think of 'older babies' as being infants that

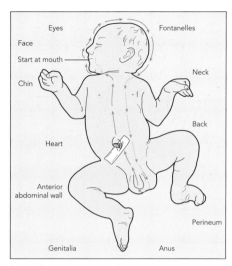

Fig. 12.5 Scheme for examining newborns. By 'circumnavigating' the baby in a systemic way, most visible congenital abnormalities will be detected. The more important congenital anomalies tend to occur on or near the midline, so using a constant point of origin (e.g. the mouth) start examining the neonate along the midline, circumnavigating the entire baby and arriving back at your point of origin. At some points you may stray from the midline (e.g. to look at the eyes, or auscultate the heart). At the end do not forget the hands, feet and hips need checking.

are not yet walking and 'toddlers' as babies who have only recently acquired this skill. The child progresses from being primarily supine and unable to move around, to becoming a toddler who is able to run and talk.

At the beginning of this period the effects of passively acquired maternal immunity (transplacental immunoglobulin G) mean that babies are not as prone to intercurrent viral illnesses as they will be later. On average, the healthy older baby and toddler will have to deal with eight self-limiting viral illnesses per year. Sometimes two or three of these illnesses will occur 'back to back', causing a great deal of anxiety in the parents, and the infant may temporarily fail to thrive.

In many developed countries, a comprehensive immunisation programme from birth to 2 years aims to prevent up to nine or more important infectious diseases (e.g. diphtheria, tetanus, pertussis, polio, *Haemophilus* type B infections, meningococcal group C infections, measles, mumps and rubella). Visits for primary immunisation provide an opportunity for the infant's primary care physician to observe an infant's growth, development and general health.

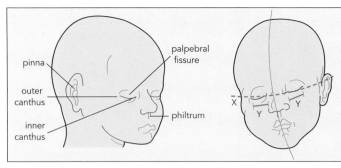

Fig. 12.6 Facial dysmorphology vocabulary explained. A few of the common anatomical terms used in describing facial features are demonstrated. The proportions of baby's face when viewed from the front, with a line through the eyes, is about half way from vertex to chin (X); the **palpebral fissures** (the slits through which your eyes look) should be of equal length (Y), measured from inner to outer **canthus**. There is usually a very mild slant to the palpebral fissures, if this slant is exaggerated then it is described as **upward slanting** (as may be seen in trisomy 21, Down's syndrome). Alternatively, the slant may be in the opposite direction and is described as **downward slanting** (as may be seen in many syndromes). The distance between the eyes is approximately that of the palpebral fissures (Y). **Hypotelorism** is when this distance is too short and **hypertelorism** is when this distance is too long and the eyes appear too far apart. The **philtrum** leads from the nostrils to the edge of the upper lip. A line from the outer canthus towards the occiput should cross the attachment of the upper helix of the **pinna** (ear lobe) to the side of the head. Where this does not occur then the ear is described as **low set** and may appear **simple** (poorly formed helix) and **rotated** as well.

Growth

The 'average infant' will have doubled birth weight by approximately 5 months and trebled it by just after a year.

The most dramatic changes are seen in head growth as a result of myelination of cortical tracts and pathways leading to rapid brain growth.

Development

At the beginning of this phase, a baby's cortical function has only recently demonstrated the important milestone of social smiling (6–8 weeks age). By the end of this phase (aged 2 years) the child will be walking, communicating wants and needs verbally and nonverbally and have developed sophisticated hand function and coordination.

The key question in this age group is: *Are the parents concerned about their child's developmental progress?*

The first areas to develop rapidly are vision and the control of hand movements and the next are the gross locomotor skills needed to roll over and sit without support. During this time visual acuity and hand dexterity are continuing to improve. Fine and gross motor development rely heavily on the progression of visual development. The child listens to adults and siblings intently. He or she starts to babble and to understand more and more of what is said. Once confidence is gained when prone with hip flexed, the baby finds him or herself teetering on hands and knees and then begins to crawl. Soon after that, the toddler is pulling up to stand and cruising around the furniture: the prelude to solo walking. Fine motor skills include the continued refinement of grasp until the pincer grip is achieved. At around the same time, vocalisations have become more and more specific and 'dada' and 'mama' are said with meaning. Comprehension of language now includes following some instructions and commands. This is all usually achieved in the first year.

In the following year, continued improvements in walking are followed by running at speed, kicking a ball and rapid changes in direction. Fine motor skills are seen in manual dexterity (tower of six cubes) and improved self-help abilities (feeding with a spoon, drinking from a cup and beginning to undress themselves). Communication continues to advance with the increase in vocabulary and the combination of words to make short phrases. Comprehension of language is still greater than expressive language abilities.

History

The history should cover the same areas as with the newborn and very young baby and include points particularly relevant to this period; for example, current feeding, weaning, developmental abilities, immunisations received.

Examination

During the history it is often best to keep the child on the parent's lap and play with him or her.

It is important, as with newborns, to examine the most relevant system indicated by the history first because this may be your only chance. Make sure that you have examined the whole child undressed by the end of your examination. This should be done in stages. Save the more unpleasant parts of the examination (e.g. looking at the ears and throat) until last.

CIRCULATION AND CARDIOVASCULAR SYSTEM

Look at the child's colour. Infants are now no longer polycythaemic; indeed they are likely to be 'physiologically' anaemic (lower end of

> Review
> **Measuring children's blood pressure**
>
> Children's blood pressure measurements can be obtained using:
> - Oscillometry (dynamap)
> - Sphygmomanometry (using a stethoscope or Doppler probe or by palpation)
> - Direct (invasive) measurement (in intensive care)
>
> Remember the two-thirds rule:
> - Cuff width must be at least two-thirds of the distance from shoulder to elbow
> - Cuff (bladder) length must be at least two-thirds of the limb circumference

expected range for haemoglobin is 9.4 g/dl at 2 months and 11.1 g/dl at 6 months).

Capillary refill time is a very sensitive sign and should be the same as for adults (less than 2–3 s). Tachycardia is an important physical sign that needs evaluation, e.g. febrile, unwell, upset and crying.

Blood pressure should be measured in any sick infant. Interpretation of a single blood pressure measurement requires knowledge of three factors: what size of cuff was used relative to the child's upper arm; the size of the child; and what emotional state the child was in at the time of measurement. The cuff size is critical, as blood pressure measurements may be spuriously high if too small a cuff is used or the infant is crying. Normal ranges are published according to size and age.

Palpation of the apex beat is helpful because some murmurs may be palpable as heaves or thrills. During auscultation of the heart sounds, normal splitting of the second heart sound may be difficult to hear in a tachycardic child.

Nearly one-third of children will have a murmur heard at some point of their lives. Less than 1% of children will have a structural heart lesion. Innocent murmurs have particular characteristics: ejection systolic flow murmurs are either 'short and buzzing' or 'soft and blowing'; venous hums are low pitched and more noticeable after exertion of inspiration and they are abolished by lying supine.

True pathological murmurs are usually louder, harsher and longer and may radiate or have a diastolic component.

BREATHING AND RESPIRATION

Watching and listening to the child's respiratory pattern is the most useful part of the examination of the respiratory system. Auscultation may add some more information, but is frequently 'drowned' by loud transmitted upper respiratory tract breath sounds.

Differential diagnosis
Nonblanching (purpuric) rashes

Rashes in childhood are very common and all you need is a simple and logical approach to make a diagnosis most of the time.

- The most clinically important rashes to recognise promptly are ones that are purpuric (nonblanching), for example, meningococcal septicaemia (Fig. 12.7), idiopathic thrombocytopenic purpura (Fig. 12.8), fingertip bruises in nonaccidental injury (Fig. 12.9) and Henoch–Schönlein purpura (Fig. 12.10).
- If the rash is erythematous (blanching) and is associated with an intercurrent illness, then it is most probably related to an infection: often viral and self-limiting
- Any chronically itchy rash is likely to be eczema and should be treated with emollients

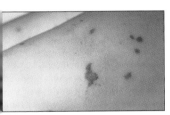

Fig. 12.7 Purpuric rashes: meningococcal septicaemia. All purpuric rashes in childhood need careful evaluation. The lives of patients with meningococcal disease depend on their doctor recognising this purpuric rash as early as possible. Note that the rash may start off as erythematous and then progress to nonblanching purpura. It is the speed of the rash's progression and the patient's degree of illness that are the hallmarks of this infection. Treat immediately with an appropriate parenteral antibiotic.

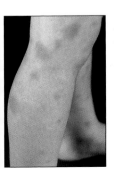

Fig. 12.8 Purpuric rashes: idiopathic thrombocytopenic purpura (ITP). ITP in childhood difffers from the adult condition by being more benign and is self-limiting. Acute leukaemia is a very important differential diagnosis to be rapidly excluded by a full blood count and blood film.

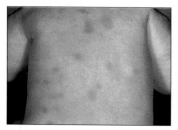

Fig. 12.9 Purpuric rashes: fingertip bruising; nonaccidental injury. All children have falls and minor injuries that result in bruises. Most bruises occur in areas of likely accidental impact (e.g. shins and elbows). Any bruise in a usually protected site is a worry. Ask how it happened. Is the injury consistent with the history? If you are worried discuss immediately with senior staff.

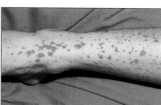

Fig. 12.10 Purpuric rashes: Henoch–Schönlein purpura (HSP). HSP is an 'allergic' vasculitis that has a characteristic distribution along the back of the legs, extending up to the buttocks. It is associated with many systemic symptoms, such as joint swelling and (uncommonly) may result in permanent renal impairment.

Look at the upper respiratory tract (in the ears, nose and throat) at the end of the examination. Coryza and pink inflamed mucous membranes in the throat and ears are most likely to be caused by a viral upper respiratory infection.

Acutely tender lymphadenopathy can be associated with bacterial infections. Persisting, asymmetrical large and nontender lymphadenopathy in association with constitutional symptoms needs accurate diagnosis.

ABDOMEN

Bile-stained vomiting, pallor, excessive inconsolable crying, a distended abdomen, lumps in the groin and blood in the stool are all indicators of an acute abdominal problem. Children with peritonitis will lie very still, with their knees flexed, and breathe without moving the diaphragm.

Palpation can be attempted with warm hands. More than one attempt at palpation may be required, perhaps when the child is sleeping on a parent's lap.

In boys, always check that the testes are in the scrotum. Do not attempt to retract the foreskin. In girls the external genitalia are less visible than when they are newborn. The labia majora are fleshy and obscure the introitus, clitoris and urethral opening.

NEUROLOGY AND DEVELOPMENT

The history is the key in many neurological diagnoses. With possible fits or 'funny turns', a first-hand account is best of all; a parent's video of the episode may be most valuable. Observation is more important than testing reflexes.

Observation of gross motor skills will enable posture, power and, when the child is picked up, tone to be assessed. In younger babies antigravity power should be demonstrable by lifting the limbs, or, when prone, the head off the bed. The limbs can be inspected and palpated in play to ascertain tone, muscle bulk, power and sensation (by gently tickling). Deep tendon reflexes can be elicited with patience. In an easily distracted child, reinforcement can be employed in play (squeeze the toy). Coordination is hard to test formally and the observation of fine motor skills and gait are the most one can rely on.

The cranial nerves can be assessed by observation of behaviour and facial expression.

The olfactory (first) nerve   This is rarely tested.

The optic (second) nerve   Examining the visual fields and employing fundoscopy is often difficult in this age group. In the older (preschool age) child this is more straightforward and acuity can be checked beyond the age of 2 years with shape or letter matching.

The oculomotor, trochlear and abducens (third, fourth and sixth) nerves   Eye movements can be observed when the child follows a toy or light in the vertical and horizontal plane.

The trigeminal (fifth) and facial (seventh) nerves   The trigeminal nerve can be tested when the jaws are clenched on a bottle or biscuit, and the facial nerve by encouraging the child to smile or shut their eyes.

The acoustic (eighth) nerve   Many places have now introduced universal Oto-Acoustic Emission (OAE) Hearing Screening in the neonatal period.

The glossopharyngeal (ninth), vagus (Xth) accessory (XIth) and hypoglossal (XIIth) nerves   A history of regurgitation or choking on feeds may be relevant.

When inspecting the throat you may be lucky and notice the following: movement of the uvula as you inspect the throat (ninth nerve intact); no hoarseness in the cry (Xth nerve intact); shrugging of the shoulders and turning of the head using the sternomastoid (XIth nerve intact); waggling of the tongue as the spatula is used (XIIth nerve intact).

THE PRESCHOOL CHILD

The preschool age group, from 2 to 5 years of age, are frequent attenders of their doctors.

Growth

Growth during this phase appears almost linear on the growth chart. The growth rate is decelerating by approximately 30% over this period.

Development

This period is characterised by advances in communication and the use and understanding of language. The advances in language, speech and communication mean that certain tests and facets of the clinical examination are approaching those used in adults.

History

The history should include details about developmental skills acquired and whether the parents or health visitor have any concerns. Other specific points include diet (peak age for incidence of dietary iron-deficiency anaemia), exercise tolerance and coughing (asthma is commonly underdiagnosed).

Examination

Generally this is best done on the parent's lap. Focus on the area of interest first and save the less pleasant parts until last. Make a game of it all and satisfy any curiosity expressed by the child (e.g. by letting them listen to mummy's heart or look in daddy's ear).

CIRCULATION AND CARDIOVASCULAR SYSTEM
The fall in heart rate means that the first and second heart sounds can be more carefully assessed. Innocent, benign flow-related murmurs are also common in this age group.

BREATHING AND RESPIRATION
Observation of the chest shape and respiratory pattern are again invaluable. Auscultation is seldom rewarding in the absence of observed respiratory distress. Peak flow measurements are not reproducible until age 4–5 years.

ABDOMEN
If the child is on a bed or couch it is important to make sure that a parent is near the head end. It is worthwhile kneeling down, making

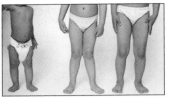

Fig. 12.11 Three boys' legs; which legs are normal? These three brothers all have normal legs. The youngest has mild genu varus (bow legs), which is physiological in the toddler. The middle brother has genu valgus (knock knees), which is physiological in the preschool-aged child. The eldest brother has 'straight' legs.

sure that the child's eye level is above yours and looking at the child's face, not the belly. It is likely that an abdominal examination will be successful.

Leg posture and gait are a frequent source of parental anxiety. Genu varus (bow legs) are normal early on; there is then a tendency to genu valgus (knock knees) before a more straight leg grows in school-age children (Fig. 12.11).

NEUROLOGY AND DEVELOPMENT

Gait and gross motor abilities are assessed as the child is playing in the room. Fine motor abilities can now be readily assessed with a pencil and paper, by asking the child to copy various shapes: a circle by age 3 years, a cross by 4 years, a square by 4 years 6 months and triangles by 5 years. Hearing can be checked using free field audiometry. Vision can be tested with shape- or letter-matching by the age of approximately 3 years.

Reflexes, fundoscopy, visual fields and specific motor and coordination tasks are all possible, as long as the child perceives your examination as fun.

THE SCHOOL-AGED CHILD

The school-age group, from 5 to 10+ years of age (until the onset of puberty), are seen less often by their doctors. It is also the age at which psychological factors are beginning to play a bigger role in how and what the child may complain of to their parents and doctors.

Growth

The height will usually be following near the midparental centile. Accelerations in height velocity may be attributed to an excessive weight gain. Decelerations may be due to inadequately managed or unrecognised chronic illness (e.g. asthma or coeliac disease) or endocrine problems.

Development

These children will become more independent from their parents and carers but more dependent on their peer group. Language and cognitive skills, literacy and numeracy are further developed in class and at home. Vision, hearing and motor skills are approaching adult abilities.

History

Invite the child to be the historian and rely on the parent for back-up. It is important to pitch the questions in terms the child understands.

Information about the home and especially school is important. Hobbies, sports and pastimes give other clues to the seriousness of the illness and its impact on the child's life.

Examination

The sequence of the examination is now more or less dictated by you. There are very few differences in technique from examining adults, except that the examination should continue to be fun.

ADOLESCENTS

- Adolescents seldom consult their doctor.
- Adolescents are in the transition from childhood to adulthood and are uncertain as to how to behave as adults.
- Doctors need to allow them to be adolescent and accept that the adolescent is easily embarrassed and often anxious.
- The presenting problems can have a psychological basis.
- Adolescents with a chronic illness will demonstrate normal adolescent rebellion, which can have long-term health consequences.
- Risk-taking behaviour (cigarettes, alcohol, drugs, sex, etc.) is normal and when it does go wrong, in health terms, it is hard not to appear judgemental and authoritative as the doctor.
- Deliberate self-harm (overdoses especially) in adolescents is becoming more prevalent.
- Confidentiality and consent are sometimes a source of conflict between patient, parent and doctor.

The adolescent's doctor needs to be open-minded about the nature and cause of the complaint and sensitive to the patient's need to be seen with (or without) a parent.

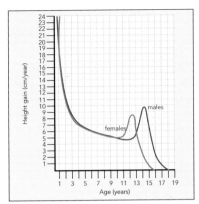

Fig. 12.12 Height velocity in girls and boys. Note how before the pubertal growth spurt there is little difference in girls' and boys' height velocities. Also note that girls' pubertal height velocity peaks are earlier and less tall than those for boys. These are thought to be the main factors determining the difference in adult male and female height.

Growth

During the first 10 years there is remarkably little difference between the height and weight velocity in the growth of girls and boys until puberty, then there is a growth spurt that lasts for 2–3 years (Fig. 12.12).

Puberty

The onset of puberty is less than 1 year apart in girls (mean age 11.4 years) and boys (mean age 12.0 years) but the pubertal growth spurt occurs in girls approximately 2 years before boys. The first physical sign of puberty in a girl is the development of breast tissue under the nipples (mean age 11 years); the first physical sign in boys is the enlargement of the testes from their prepubertal volume of less than 2 ml to an endocrinologically active volume of greater than 4 ml (mean age 12 years).

A constitutional delay in growth and puberty is more of a problem for boys than girls because boys have their pubertal growth spurt 2 years later than girls and because boys' growth spurts are larger than girls', so its absence is more apparent.

In girls, when the growth spurt (height velocity) decelerates to less than 4 cm per year, the menarche can occur; height continues to increase for 1.5–2 years after the menarche. Final adult height is achieved

> **D$_x$** Differential diagnosis
> **Constitutional delay in growth and puberty**
>
> - This condition is most common in boys
> - Patients usually have a history of growing in the lower quartile of the normal range but by the middle teenage years are very much shorter than their peers (at this time they present to a specialist clinic)
> - Severe psychological stress may result from this genetic and physiological delay in puberty
> - Pharmacologically inducing puberty is an effective way of relieving the stress suffered by these patients

when the bony epiphyses fuse in the vertebrae and along the long bones of the leg.

Development

Development continues long after growth has finished. It is mostly in the spheres of social and behavioural development that adolescents are still progressing.

The gap between the end of growth and the end of development into a fully independent adult is apparently widening. The mean age for pubertal milestones appears to have come down from that of a century ago.

History

Depending on the presenting problem, it may be necessary to agree who remains in the consulting room. This is one area in which confidentiality and consent may become a point of conflict. It is important to direct your questions primarily to the patient, and only when necessary to the parent or carer.

Details about the family and relationships between members of the household are important. Details about school, progress with school work, hobbies, sports, pastimes and friendships can all help give an indication of how the adolescent is coping with the increasing stresses of the real world.

Examination

Most adolescents are very self-conscious of their appearance, so make sure they have suitable facilities (e.g. blankets and screens around the examination couch). The examining doctor will need to decide during the history-taking whether the parent is to be invited alongside the patient. When an adolescent is seen alone during the physical examination, it is advisable to include a chaperone in the examination room.

Apart from the assessment of growth and puberty and attention to the adolescent and parent relationship, the rest of the examination will be similar to that for an adult patient.

Review
Child development

This is a difficult subject to summarise because of the large degree of normal variation in acquisition of skills (milestones). Always correct age for prematurity. Some warning signs in the first year of life include:

- Any child whose parent expresses specific concerns about his or her development
- The loss of any acquired skills (developmental regression)
- Persistence of adducted thumbs from the neonatal period
- No social smile by age 8 weeks
- No startling to sound or responding to nearby voices by 8 weeks
- Not visually fixing and following from before 8 weeks
- Definite asymmetry of tone and movement (with head in midline) during the first year
- Not sitting unsupported by 8 months
- No polysyllabic babbling by 8 months